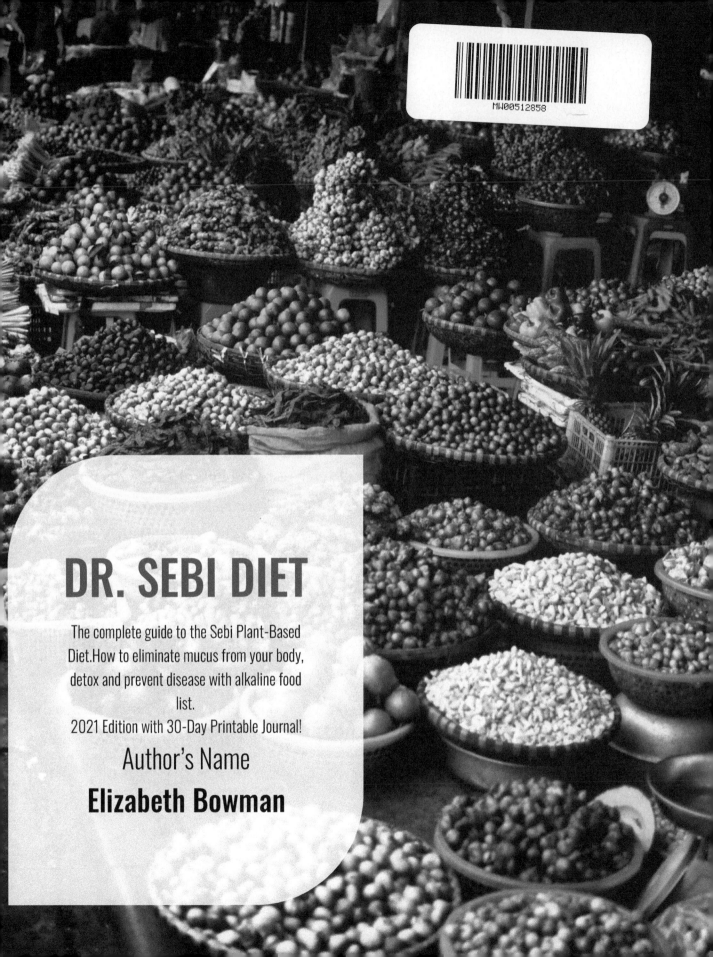

DR. SEBI DIET

The complete guide to the Sebi Plant-Based
Diet.How to eliminate mucus from your body,
detox and prevent disease with alkaline food
list.
2021 Edition with 30-Day Printable Journal!

Author's Name

Elizabeth Bowman

THIS BOOK INCLUDES

The diary

Dr. Sebi Journal

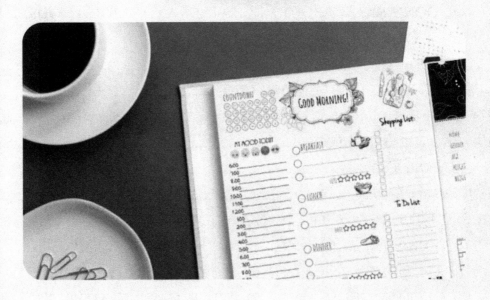

FILLABLE AND PRINTABLE ONLINE VERSION!!!

THE FOOD AND MOTIVATIONAL DIARY, MADE EXCLUSIVELY FOR THIS BOOK

TABLE OF CONTENTS

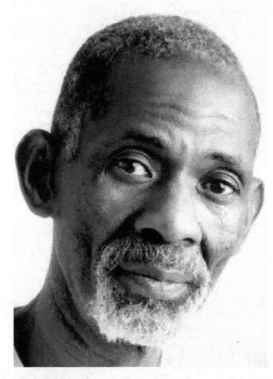

*"If nature didn't make it,
Don't take it!"*

Dr. Alfredo "Sebi" Bowman

INTRODUCTION

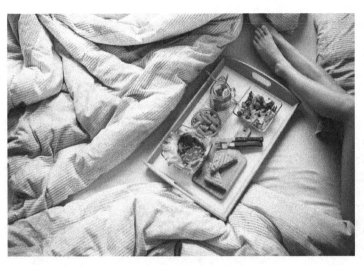

It is just recently that an ever-increasing number of individuals are beginning to embrace the plant-based diet way of life. With respect to what precisely has drawn a huge number of individuals into this way of life is disputable. Nonetheless, there is developing proof showing that after a fundamentally plant-based diet way of living prompts better weight control and general wellbeing, liberated from numerous constant sicknesses. This book will take you through the rudiments of this way of life, its advantages, and why it works, as well as gives you thoughts on how you can patch up your storeroom and begin preparing heavenly plant-based dishes and other diets suggested by Dr. Sebi. Regardless of whether you are new to this way of life or accustomed to it, this book is unquestionably a fortune.

PART ONE
CHAPTER 1

BRIEF HISTORY OF DOCTOR SEBI

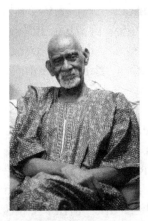

Dr. Sebi is a pathologist, herbalist, organic biochemist, and naturalist. He has personally observed herbs and studied leaves in different continents across the globe such as in Central, South and North America, Africa, and the Caribbean.

Dr. Sebi had developed a fascinating procedure and methodology of healing the human body system with herbs and roots that are solidly established in more than 30 years of research and involvement.

DR. SEBI'S EARLY BIRTH

Dr. Sebi was born Bowman Alfredo on November 26, 1933, in Ilanga in Spanish Honduras. He is a self-learned physician. He learned at the foot of his cherished grandmother, "Mama Hay." Neither formal physician training in medical doctor nor did he hold a Ph.D., but his early days of knowledge and observation by the waterline area and the woodlands, joined with bearings from his grandmother, overseen Sebi the foundation to be faithful in his career.

MIGRATION TO THE WESTERN WORLD AND HIS WORKS

Dr. Sebi migrated to the United States as a self-educated man diagnosed with asthma, diabetes, impotence, and obesity. After unsuccessful treatments with conventional doctors and traditional western medicine, Sebi led to an herbalist in Mexico. Finding great healing success from all his ailments, he began creating natural vegetation cell food compounds geared for inter-cellular cleansing and revitalizing all the cells that make up the human body. Dr. Sebi has dedicated decades of his life to developing a unique methodology that he could only obtain through years of empirical knowledge.

Inspired by the personal healing experience and knowledge he gained, he began sharing the compounds with others, giving birth to Dr. Sebi's Cell Food website. As shown by Health Line, he initially communicated that his herbs could fix chronic conditions, for instance, AIDS, sickle cell anemia, and lupus. Nevertheless, in 1987, he was caught for practicing drug without a license (notwithstanding the way that the jury vindicated him). A few years later, after another case by the State of New York, Sebi agreed to stop making claims that his products could cure any sicknesses.

STORIES BEHIND HIS DEATH

Although controversial, Dr. Sebi's list of clients included: Michael Jackson, John Travolta, and Steven Seagal. Sebi was later arrested in 2016 for money laundering. While jailed in Honduras, he contracted pneumonia and died on the way to the hospital.

Despite the fact that he is deceased, his discoveries and self-invention on mucus cures and diets are still helping millions of patients worldwide. During his time on earth, Dr. Sebi healed millions of mucus individuals with his diet method, and his death has done little to change this. He left behind holistic healing for hair loss. You can learn from his life and what he believed about this deadly disease to eradicate mucus from the surface of the earth; here are the complete analysis of Dr. Sebi's cure for healing is all about and his plans of diets.

CHAPTER 2

DIET

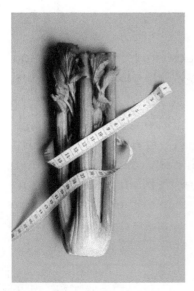

Hearing the word "diet" makes us think of an unpleasant weight-loss meal? If it did, you are doubtless not alone in this assumption. For example, consider using the words "Diet" in marketing food products and supplements—it usually explains foods small in calories. But in scientific terms and definitions, Diet *can also refer to the food and drink people consume daily and the mental and physical circumstances connected to eating.* Nutrition involves more than merely eating appropriate diets—it is about nourishment on every food intake and treatment of our body's ailments, our community, and the world. A balanced diet can also involve the occasional treat, and it should be enjoyed; after all, everyone needs something one day. In the end, you will feel better about yourself but not only that you will probably burn a lot of fat!

WHAT IS DR. SEBI BELIEVES ON DIET

Dr. Sebi claims that illness is a consequence of Pus, mucus, and corrosiveness in the body and contended that sicknesses couldn't exist in an antacid climate or alkaline environment. His program, which incorporates severe dietary routine and costly supplements, claims to detoxify the infection group and reestablish alkalinity. The diet restricts dairy products of any kind and overall focuses on the vegan diet, yet with many stricter principles. For instance, it restricts seedless fruits and only permits Sebi's approved list of "natural growing grains."

All nourishments or foods that are pus/mucus-forming are corrosive in nature. "Acid" is from the mid-1600s signifying "of the taste of vinegar," from French acid (16c.) or straightforwardly from Latin acidus "harsh, sour sharp," modifier of state from acere "to be sour," from PIE root *ak-"sharp, pointed" (see acrid). In chemistry, it alludes to a class of substances whose solution arrangements are described by an acrid taste, the capacity to turn blue litmus red, and the capacity to respond with bases and certain metals to form salts. From a mucusless point of view, pus and mucus-forming nourishments are perceived to be "corrosive framing" inside the human body. Such nourishments establish an acidic inner environment that is inconvenient to health and detrimental to wellness.

WHAT YOU DON'T KNOW ABOUT MUCUS, PLUS AND ACIDIC FOODS

The word "mucus" is from the Latin tongue language, which indicates "mold, snot, slime, etc." Mucus refers to dense, thick, slippery discharges comprised of dead cells, mucin, inorganic substances, and exfoliated cells. Also refers to slimy, sticky, viscous substance left behind by mucus-forming foods in the body after intake. While the antonyms word "mucusless," or mucus-free, refers to substances or foods that are not mucus-composed such intakes digest without leaving behind mucus. These foods include all likes of fat-free and starchless fruits and vegetables. While "Pus" is from late 14c. Latin "Pus" (identified with puter [putrid] "spoiled") from Proto-Indo-European*pu-contrasted with Sanskrit. Puyat "spoils, smells," Putih "smelling, foul." Pus frequently alludes to a thick white, yellowish or greenish opaque liquid produced in infected tissue, comprising dead white platelets or white blood cells, microscopic organisms, tissue garbage, and serum. It also knows to be a substance that dead creature tissue is synthetically changed to after being devoured or while decaying in one's stomach tract. The ingestion of meat and dairy items make pus buildup in the body, while starchy and fatty nourishments are mucus-forming.

LIST OF MUCUS AND ACIDIC-FORMING FOODS

CEREALS (MODERATELY MUCUS-FORMING)

- Barley
- Pieces of bread (appreciable amount; Barley, Black, Rye, White, Graham, Pumpernickel, Zwieback, etc.)
- Cereal Grains (All Kinds of; Maize, Farina, Kamut, Millet, Oats, Quinoa, White or Brown Rice, Wheat)
- Pseudocereals Cornmeal (All Kinds; Amaranth, Buckwheat, Chia, Cockscomb, Kañiwa, Quinoa, etc.)
- Kinds of pasta.

BEANS (MODERATELY MUCUS-FORMING)

- Beans (All Kinds and Forms; Fava Beans, Butter Beans, Black Beans, Black-eyed peas, Edamame, Great Northern Beans, Italian Beans, Kidney Beans, Lentils, Lima Beans, Mung Beans, Cannellini Beans, Chickpeas/Garbanzo Beans, Navy Beans, Pinto Beans, Soya Beans, Split Peas, White Beans, String Beans, Green Beans, etc.)

NUTS AND SEEDS (MUCUS-FORMING)

- Nuts (All Kinds and forms; Acorns, Almonds, Brazil Nuts, Cashews, Chestnuts, Peanuts, Pecans, Pistachios', Walnuts, Hazelnuts, etc.)
- Seeds (All Kinds; Sunflower, Pumpkin, Hemp, Sesame, etc.)

DAIRY PRODUCTS (PUS-FORMING)

- Cow meat
- Buttermilk
- Cheese (All Kinds)
- Cream
- Crème Fraiche
- Kefir
- Butter
- Kinds of milk (All Animals and Kinds; Raw Organic, Skim, 1 or 2 %, etc.)
- Yogurts

FISH (PUS-FORMING)

- Crustacean (Crawfish, Crab, Lobster, Shrimp)
- Fish (All kinds)
- Mollusks (Oysters, Clam, Mussels, Snail, etc.)
- Roe (Caviar)
- Shell Fish
- Salmon

FLESH (PUS-FORMING)

- Blood of Animals
- Eggs (All Kinds)
- Lard
- Meat (Chicken, Beef, Goat, Dog, Lamb/Mutton, Turkey, Veal, Pork:
- Bacon, Ham, Gammon, Sausage, Chitterlings, Pig Feet; Wild Game: Bison, Buffalo, Ostrich, Rabbit, etc.)
- Margarine (Made from Animal Fat)

PROCESSED FOODS (PUS AND VERY MUCUS-FORMING)

- Dried Convenience Foods
- Fast Foods
- Packaged Convenience Foods
- Frozen Convenience Foods
- Processed Meat

CONFECTIONERIES/ CANDY (PUS AND VERY MUCUS-FORMING)

- Baked Goods (All kinds including cakes, pies, pastries, etc.)
- Candy (All Types; Bars, Caramels, Choco, Jelly candies, Rock Candy, Taffy.
- Gelatin (Jell-O)
- Ice Cream (Dairy and Non-Dairy)
- Marshmallow
- Sweets

VEGETARIAN/VEGAN PROCESSED FOODS (MODERATELY MUCUS FORMING)

- Chips (corn, potato, plantain, etc.)
- Frozen Vegan Breakfast Foods (waffles, etc.)
- Hummus (processed chickpeas)
- Lab-Grown Animal Tissue
- Margarine
- Nutritional Yeast
- Pasta (egg-free)
- Pasteurized 100% Fruit Juice (potentially acid-forming)
- Plant milk (grains, nuts, seeds, and legumes including soy, rice, etc.)
- Plant-based butter (nuts, seeds, and legumes including soy, peanut, etc.)

- Plant-based creamers
- Soy Lecithin (food additive)
- Tempeh
- Texturized Vegetable Protein ('mock' meats including soy, etc.)
- Tofu
- Vegan Baked Goods
- Vegan Confections (All Types; Chocolates, Ice Cream, etc.)
- Vegan Cheese Substitutes
- Vegan Mayonnaise
- Vegan Whipped Cream
- Yogurts (Plant-based)

ACIDIC, FERMENTED, AND DISTILLED DRINKS/SYRUPS (ACID-FORMING STIMULANTS)

- Mead, Porter, Cider, Liqueur, Rum, Sake/Rice Wine, Gin, Herbal Wine, Lager, Fruit Wine, Vodka Whisky, Tequila, etc.)
- Alcoholic Beverages (All Kinds of Beer, Ale, Brandy, Champagne, Hard drinks, etc.)
- Syrups (Barley Malt, Chocolate, Brown Rice, Corn, Artificially Flavored)
- Cocoa/Coffee
- Kombucha Tea
- Soft Drink (Soda Pop)
- Tea (All Kinds from the Theaceae family)
- Vinegar (White, Apple Cider)
- Old-fashioned Root Beer

FERMENTED FOODS AND SAUCES (ACID-FORMING STIMULANTS)

- Fish Sauce

- Fermented Vegetables (All kinds; Kimchi/cabbage and other veggies, Olives and oils.)
- Pickles/cucumbers. Sauerkraut/cabbage, etc.)
- Miso
- Sauces with Vinegar (Hot Sauce, Ketchup, Cultured and Kombucha Mustard, Mayonnaise, Relish, Tartar, Barbecue, Salad Dressings, Salsa, etc.)
- Soy Sauce
- Lacto-fermented Homemade Mayonnaise

OILS, FATTY AND MILDLY (MUCUS FORMING)

- Oil (All types and kinds; Chia Seed, Coconut, Corn, Cotton Seed, Cotton Seed, Flax Seed, Avocado Oil, Grape Seed, Hemp Seed, Olive, Palm, Peanut, Quinoa, Nut Oils, Rapeseed, Safflower, Soybean, etc.)

SALTS AND SPICES (STIMULANTS/POTENTIALLY ACID-FORMING)

- Black Peppercorns
- Cayenne Pepper
- Chili Powder
- Cream of Tarter
- Curry Powder
- Nutmeg
- Paprika
- Pepper
- Salt (Celery, Crystal, Iodized, Sea)
- Vanilla Extract

STARCHY/FATTY VEGETABLES AND FRUITS (SLIGHTLY MUCUS-FORMING)

- Avocados
- Artichoke
- Cauliflower
- Corn
- Cassava
- Coconut Meat
- Durian
- Fungus (Mushrooms)
- Green Peas
- Olives
- Parsnips
- Peas (Raw)
- Plantain
- Plantains
- Pumpkins
- Raw or Baked White Potatoes
- Raw Squashes (Winter, Acorn, Butternut, etc.)
- Raw Sweet Potatoes
- Turnip
- Rutabaga
- Unripe Banana

WHAT ARE DECEPTIVE MUCUS-FORMERS?

Here is a rundown of nourishments that numerous individuals don't understand make mucus:

- **Rice** (extraordinary for making glue to bind books, bad for the transition to a mucus-free diet)

- **Avocados** (fatty items that might be utilized on the transition, however, are profoundly addictive. Although fruity, if used it is best to combine them with a mucus-free combination salad or vegetables to aid elimination. However, it is prescribed to avoid them on the off chance that you are not effectively adhered to them)

- **Nuts** (Mucus-forming, but may be used on transition. It is ideal to eat with dried natural products like raisins to help with disposal.)

- **Plantains** (Starchy)

- **Tofu** (Slimy and mucus-forming.)

- **Un-aged organic products like green bananas** (the riper the organic product you eat the better).

- **Corn** (It doesn't dispense well. At the point when cooked corn or corn chips are eating it gets soft and vile in the digestive organs.)

- **Corn chips** (they are exceptionally addictive and don't dispense with well)

- **Beans** (They are starchy and mucus-forming. they might be utilized sparingly on the progress inside closeness to green-verdant plates of mixed greens)

- **Starchy Vegetables** (Boring Vegetables (Some vegetables are bland and bodily fluid framing in crude or cooked structures, for example, white potatoes. Yet, numerous different vegetables, for example, yams, become nearly mucus free (starchless) after appropriate cooking.

CHAPTER 3

WEIGHT LOSS AND GOOD HEALTH

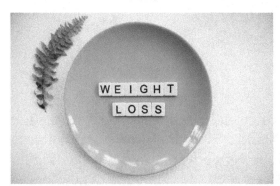

The book you are holding in your hands is a thoroughly rewritten version of Dr. Sebi's work. Having listened to and research the people who followed his weight control program, I have clarified and improved the "do-ability" of the practical section of this book. I've added many new pieces of research in history, new ways to reduced weight, and improved recipes. Finally, I have assigned information on the recent upsurge of scientific evidence and research. We had it right then, and now; we have twice as much research to confirm the nutritional approach championed by Dr. Sebi.

THE PROMISE

Lose weight! Look good! Increase energy! This section of the book will show you how it's done. Not alone, it will also show you how to change your life for the better. Thousands of famous and low profile men in history have followed its teachings and methods for decades. Most of you will have heard people with testimony saying it's the most effective weight loss program they've ever tried. Yes, it is! They've been through the weight-loss wars and conquered with this legendary approach. List them and I tell it you've probably attempted it, regardless of whether it's a low-fat diet, a food-combining diet, the grapefruit diet, fluid diets, other craze eats fewer crabs unendingly. You've figured out how to check calories, in any case with no achievement. Regardless of whether you shed pounds, you were regularly ravenous and consistently felt denied. At that point when you returned to your old method of eating, those pounds crawled back, regularly joined by a couple of something else. If this scenario sounds very familiar, I have an answer that will help end the round of yo-yo counting calories for the last time. All things being equal, I'll assist you with embracing a lasting method of eating that:

1. Let you get in shape without counting calories.

2. Makes you feel and look better.

3. Naturally re-stimulates you.

4. Keeps lost pounds off perpetually with another lifetime nourishing methodology that incorporates rich, delightful nourishments.

Be that as it may, notwithstanding weight reduction, there is a significantly more significant advantage: The wholesome approach you'll find out about here is additionally a progressive technique for living a long, solid life. I need my reader to declare: "I realized I'd lose weight; however, I never acknowledged how to feel healthier.

CHANGING YOUR MINDSET

Have you gotten an idea with the possibility that to lose weight and feel great you need to adopt a low-fat diet? Assuming this is the case, the standards and approach I'm going to outline for you might appear counterintuitive but will be very effective and outstanding. In the decade's years back when Dr. Sebi published his first research and claim, then a new logical and scientific approach has been led, conducted and published that shows that a controlled starch healthful methodology is better for you and your body than a low fat, high-starch nourishing methodology. But let's quit wasting time. Here are three inquiries you ought to present yourself directly:

- **Is this safe**? Indeed, and there is a lot of hard science to back that up. Truth be told, various investigations directed in the previous years (which we will allude to in future sections) show that a controlled sugar dietary methodology improves the clinical boundaries influencing coronary illness and different diseases while not causing harm to your liver, kidneys or bone structure.

- **Is this healthfully solid**? Yes, an individual after consuming the regular menu and eating nourishments containing only 20 grams of carbohydrates or surpasses the day-by-day recommended amount of most vitamins, nutrients, and minerals. As you move through the phase of Dr. Sebi, you get much more. What's better, not as indicated by me but accepted by world well-known organizations and used by most of the practicing nutritionists.

- **Will I keep off all the shed pounds?** Nothing could be all the more obvious. Whenever you've seen the outcomes and conceded to great wellbeing, you'll understand that it's a lot simpler than you ever suspected conceivable. In view of the sorts of nourishments that are essential, it's really conceivable to joyfully roll out an improvement in the manner you eat, look and feel good.

THE FOUR PRINCIPLE OF DR. SEBI NUTRITIONAL APPROACH ON WEIGH LOSS

Following the Dr. Sebi Nutritional Approach for weight, you will achieve four things:

YOU WILL GET IN SHAPE

It's hard not to. Either male or female everyone who follows Dr. Sebi's way to deal with weight reduction promptly takes off pounds and inches. For the little numbers who have no metabolic protection from weight reduction, subsequent sections will broadly expand on the best way to defeat the hindrances that forestall a fruitful result. Streamlining body weight is an important component of any wellbeing focused program in light of the fact that, all around, being essentially overweight is a marker of potential medical conditions, in the present or later on. At the point when you've taken the pounds off, you'll see the advantages, and they will be definitely more than only corrective.

YOU WILL KEEP UP YOUR WEIGHT REDUCTION

This is the place where Dr. Sebi's Nutritional Approach leaves other weight control plans in the dust. Pretty much every accomplished calorie counter has started eating less, buckled down, lost a ton of pounds, and restored them all in a couple of months or maybe a year. This is typical because of the normal result of low-fat/low-calorie counts of calories hunger. Although numerous individuals can endure hunger for some time, not many can endure it for a lifetime. Hardship is unpleasant. When the organic hole among yearning and satisfaction becomes excessively big, the bounce-back can be incredibly fast, just as tragic and mortifying. However, that is the issue of diets that confine amounts. This kind of approach won't acknowledge hunger as a lifestyle. The arrangement incorporates nourishments that have enough fat and protein so hunger isn't the big issue it is on other weight reduction plans. Be that as it may, it actually permits calorie counters to keep up a sound load for a lifetime.

YOU WILL ACCOMPLISH GREAT WELLBEING

The change is astounding. Doing Dr. Sebi's approach, you meet your wholesome needs by eating tasty, sound, filling nourishments and dodging the sugar and carbs that lousy nourishment is stacked with. Subsequently, you become not so much drained but rather more vivacious, not only in light of the weight reduction but since the physical results of really useless glucose and insulin digestion are turned around. Secondly, individuals begin feeling great even before they arrive at their objective weight. When they surrender the calamitous American eating regimen of refined sugars for entire, crude food, they begin to live once more.

It's one of the most compensating encounters I've had the benefit of seeing with a large number of my patients.

YOU WILL LAY THE PERPETUAL FOUNDATION FOR INFECTION COUNTERACTION

This will transform you, which, in all honesty, is much more significant than looking great on the seashore the following summer. By following an individualized controlled carbohydrate dietary methodology that outcomes in lower insulin creation, individuals at high danger for persistent sicknesses, for example, cardiovascular illness, hypertension, and diabetes will see a stamped improvement in their clinical measures. We will investigate a considerable lot of the researches referred to here all through the later sections of this book.

WHY CHOOSE DR. SEBI'S NUTRITIONAL APPROACH

The obvious fact is that millions of individuals don't eat the kinds of nourishments that give a steady healthy metabolism. Humanity isn't equipped to deal with a bounty of refined sugars. Getting more fit doesn't involve tallying calories; it involves eating food your body can deal with. Let me place a couple of realities on the table, all of which we will investigate all through the rest of this book:

- Most obesity came into play when the body's digestion or metabolism cycle by which it transforms food into energy, isn't functioning accurately. The more overweight an individual is, the more certain is the presence of metabolic unsettling influence.

- The foundation of the metabolic aggravation in heftiness doesn't have to do with the fat you eat. It has to do with eating an excessive amount of carbohydrate, which prompts metabolic issues, for example, insulin obstruction and hyper insulin. Furthermore, these metabolic issues are legitimately identified with your overall wellbeing picture and your probability of being misled by executioners such as diabetes, coronary illness, heart disease, and stroke. Additionally, high insulin levels have been related to a higher rate of diabetes.

- The metabolic effect also sources from excess insulin produced in the body which can be circumvented by a controlled sugary diet. Avoid the foods that cause you to be fat by controlling your intake of refined carbohydrates.

- This metabolic adjustment is striking to such an extent that some of us will have the option to lose weight by eating a higher number of calories than you've been eating on diets top-heavy unbalanced in sugars.

- Diets high in sugars are correctly what most overweight individuals don't require and can't turn out to be forever slim on. Low-fat weight control plans are, by their very nature, quite often rich-carbohydrate diets less and welcome on the very issues that they were expected to shield us from.

- Our pandemics of diabetes, coronary illness, and hypertension are to a great extent the adamant effects of our overconsumption of refined starches and its association with hyperinsulinism.

DIFFERENT KINDS OF FOODS

- *Protein* is a complex chain of amino acids-is the fundamental structure block of life and basic to pretty much every synthetic response in the human body. Food wealthy in protein incorporates meat, fish, fowl, eggs-the greater part of which contain basically no carbohydrates-and cheese, nuts, and seeds. Numerous vegetables are additionally all around provided, however dissimilar to other animal's foods, don't contain all the fundamental amino acids.

- *Fat* gives glycerol and basic unsaturated fat called fatty acids, which the body can't produce on its own. Fat is found in fish, fowl, meat, dairy items, and the oils got from nuts and seeds and a couple of vegetables, for example, avocados. Oils separated from these nourishments signify 100 percent fat and contain no carbohydrates.

- *Carbohydrate* incorporates sugars and starches that are chains of sugar particles. Despite the fact that carbohydrate gives the snappiest source of energy, we eat substantially more of it, by a wide margin, than our body should be healthy. Vegetables do contain a few starches; however, they likewise contain a wide and wondrous variety of nutrients and minerals. Notwithstanding, you can eat a lot of vegetables with high groupings of useful supplements and still control your junk. Then again, starches, for example, those in sugar and white flour contain practically nothing that your body needs in large quantities.

WHAT DO WE DO?

If you need to be weight smart and health-wise, you can't eat as I've portrayed. But you can eat the natural, fruit and vegetable nourishments as described by Dr. Sebi. Nor do you need to eat like a bunny; you can eat like a person. You can appreciate fish, sheep, steak and lobster, nuts and berries, eggs, and spread alongside a magnificent assortment of a plate of mixed greens, a variety of salad, and different vegetables.

WHAT DO YOU EAT?

Do you accept that a man can go from gaining 0.5 pounds seven days a week to losing 3.9 pounds seven days without modifying the number of calories he consumes? Let me tell you about Harry Clark. I need you to give close consideration to his story and make an effort not to offer disbelief or incredulity because these outcomes are genuine. Harry Clark, the 40-year-old director of a lumberyard, came to me with a heart arrhythmia and a frantic weight issue. He had been chubby even as a kid, yet now things were worse and out of hand. A couple of years prior, he had gone to a low-fat eating regimen focus and had figured out how to drop from 245 to 185 pounds, Sounds great. Yet, in a little while, Harry had recovered everything with an addition of another 35 pounds. Believe it or not, when Harry came to see me, he weighed 280 on a five-foot six-and-a-half-inch outline. In the past 35 months, eating a generally bland, low-fat diet of around 2,100 calories every day, he had increased 70 pounds, precisely 2 pounds per month. Harry began Dr. Sebi's diet, radically restricting his consumption of carbohydrates while eating unreservedly meat, fish, fowl, and eggs. Harry was told he could eat as much as he expected to feel fulfilled. The carbohydrate level was strikingly like what he had been eating on his past eating regimen. A quarter of a year into his new routine, he had lost 50.5 pounds (just about 4 pounds every week), and afterward kept on losing at a consistent 3 pounds' week by week. His heart manifestations disappeared, his absolute cholesterol level dropped from a mid-range 207 to a significantly lower 134 and his fatty went from 134 to 31.

HOW TO OVERCOME CHALLENGES

- Get directly in the track again on the off chance that you sporadically "tumble off."
- Stop pigging out surprisingly fast.
- Manage desires for sweets and starches.
- Guarantee that what you lose is fat and not fit body tissue.
- Change your food decisions as indicated by your own metabolism.
- Supplement your dinners with vita nutrients to help conquer metabolic obstruction.
- With your primary care physician's supervision, wipe out specific medications that helped keep your obesity.

HOW TO GET HEALTHY

- Defeat diet-related conditions, for example, unstable blood glucose, yeast diseases, and food bigotries.

- Dodge the wellbeing calamity of hyperinsulinism.

- Improve your energy level, which will make practice simpler.

- Locate the privileged vita nutrients to supplement the nourishments you eat for complete nutrition.

- Bring down your cholesterol and fatty substance levels and improve your other blood science esteems.

- Address the ailments particularly diabetes, coronary illness, and high blood pressure so frequently connected with obesity.

HOW TO DEAL WITH THE DAY-TO-DAY ISSUES

- Explore grocery store aisles to discover controlled junks, low-sugar nourishments.

- Eat out easily in exquisite eateries or even cheap food chains.

- Attend dinner gatherings without trading off your health improvement plan or culpable your hosts.

- Clarify your better approach to eating what you love.

- Take some time off or go to uncommon capacities without cheating.

- Eat serenely with those whose style of eating remains not the same as yours.

WHAT TO EAT AND CONTROL YOUR WEIGHT GAIN

1. Exercise is beneficial for you, and it will enable you to lose. Besides, it makes you burn calories; however, it quickens your metabolism, speeding up with which each other aspect of a get- a weight loss program works and keeps you headed for better wellbeing.

2. Now we briefly discuss the meal plans according to Dr. Sebi. Follow his menu for the first week, and then repeat it for another week. The menu table below is an example of *"7-day plan detox"*

DAYS	BREAKFAST	LUNCH	DINNER
MONDAY	Blueberry Avocado Chia Smoothie And Potato	Cucumber Tomato Salad	Chewy Lemon And Oatmeal
TUESDAY	Pounded Cauliflower And Green Bean Casserole	Mushroom Salad	Fiery Vegan Black Bean
WEDNESDAY	Dairy-Free Banana Nut Muffins	Mediterranean Vegetable Spaghetti	Vegetable Salad
THURSDAY	No-Bake Sweet Potato Chocolate Chip Cookies and Cinnamon Apple Smoothie	Spinach and cheese omelet Mixed green salad	Chocolate Buckwheat Granola Bars
FRIDAY	Avocado Salad	Crude Apple Tart	Berry Basil Popsicles
SATURDAY	Chocolate Buckwheat Granola Bars	Berry Basil Popsicles	Pasta Salad
SUNDAY	One And A Half Slices Zucchini Nut Bread	Broiled cheeseburger Large mixed green salad with two tomato slices	Dairy-Free Banana Nut Muffins

CHAPTER 4

PLANT-BASED DIET

WHAT IS A PLANT-BASED DIET?

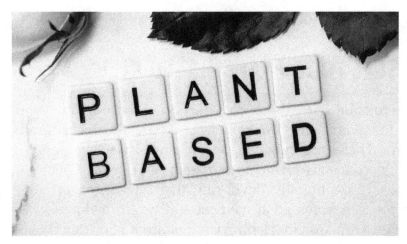

Many individuals are doing it; many people are discussing it, however, there is still a lot of disarray about what an entire food plant-based diet truly implies.

Since we break food into its macronutrients: carbohydrates, proteins, and fats; a large portion of us get befuddled about how to eat.

Imagine a scenario where we could assemble back those macronutrients again with the goal that you can free your psyche of confusion and stress. Effortlessness is the key here. Entire nourishments are natural food sources that originate from the earth. Presently, we do eat some insignificantly handled nourishment on a whole food source plant-based diet routine, for example, whole-wheat pasta, tofu, non-dairy milk, and a few nuts and seed spread.

All these mentioned categories are fine as long as they are negligibly handled. In this way, here are the various classifications:

- Whole grains Legumes (essentially lentils and beans)
- Fruits and vegetables
- Nuts and seeds (counting nut spread)
- Herbs and spices.

All the previously mentioned classifications make up an entire nourishment plant-based eating routine. Where the pleasant comes in is the way you set them up; how you season and cook them; and how you blend and match to give them extraordinary flavor and assortment in your suppers. There are sections in this book devoted to the advantages of plant-based diets which can give you a thought of what you can prepare genuine fast in your kitchen or those uncommon suppers you can get ready for the family. However long you are eating nourishments like these consistently, you can disregard junk, protein, and fat until the end of time.

Because you have settled on the choice to adopt a plant-based diet way of life, doesn't imply that is a healthy diet. Plant-based eating regimens have something reasonable of garbage and other unhealthy eats; case and point, ordinary consumption of veggie pizzas and non-dairy frozen yogurt. Remaining healthy expects you to eat good and balanced nourishments– even inside a plant-based diet setting

GETTING STARTED ON A WHOLE FOOD PLANT-BASED DIET

A typical misconception among numerous individuals– even a portion of those in the health and fitness industry is that any individual who changes to a plant-based diet routine naturally turns out to be excessively healthy. There are huge loads of plant-based low-quality nourishments out there, for example, non-dairy ice cream and frozen veggie pizza, which can truly derail your health goals if you are continually devouring them. Focusing on solid nourishments is the main way that you can accomplish medical and health benefits. Then again, these plant-based bites do assume a function in keeping you inspired. They ought to be devoured in moderation, sparingly, and in little pieces. As you will come to see later on in this book, there is a section committed to giving thoughts on plant-based snacks you can prepare at home. Thus, right away, this is how you get started on a whole food plant-based recipe.

DECIDE WHAT A PLANT-BASED DIET MEANS FOR YOU

Making a choice to structure how your plant-based diet will look is the initial step, and it will assist you with changing from your present diet standpoint. This is something that is truly personal and varies from one individual to the next. While a few people conclude that they won't endure any animal products at all, some manage with smidgens of dairy or meat occasionally. It is truly dependent upon you to choose what and how you need your plant-based eating routine to resemble. Interestingly, entire plant-based nourishments need to make an incredible lion's share of your eating diet as describe by Dr. Sebi.

COMPREHEND WHAT YOU ARE EATING ALL RIGHT

Now you've got the decision part down, your next assignment will include a lot of analysis on your part.? Indeed, if this is your first time evaluating the plant-based eating routine, you might be astonished by the number of nourishments, particularly packaged food sources, which contain animal products. You will end up supporting the propensity for understanding names while you are shopping. Turns out, heaps of prepackaged nourishments have animal products in them, so in the event that you need to adhere just to plant products for your new diet routine, you'll have to watch out for ingredient labels. Maybe you decided to permit some measure of animal products in your diet; well, you are still going to watch out for nourishments stacked with fats, sugars, sodium, additives, and different things that might affect your healthy diet.

FIND REVAMPED VERSIONS OF YOUR FAVORITE RECIPES

I'm certain you have various most loved dishes that are not really plant-based. For the vast majority, abandoning all that is generally the hardest part. Nonetheless, there is yet a way you could meet midway. Set aside some effort to consider what you like about those non-plant-based suppers. Think along the lines of flavor, texture, adaptability, etc.; and search for trades in the entire food plant-based eating routine that can satisfy what you will be missing. Just to give you some understanding of what I mean, here are a few models: Crumbled or mixed tofu would make for a decent filling in both sweet and appetizing dishes simply like ricotta cheddar would in lasagna. Lentils go especially well with saucy dishes that are commonly connected with meatloaf and Bolognese.

ALKALINE PLANT DIET

We have to change the Western eating routine, which is being globalized, from being fixed on meat, dairy, processed foods, and hybridized and hereditarily changed plant nourishments, to a diet that is focused on the consumption of alkaline plant foods. We should look to the plant nourishments that are indigenous to Africa or different zones of the world that share the equivalent or comparative ecological state and environmental conditions of Africa, similar to Central and South America, the Caribbean, and India. These foods develop under similar conditions that upheld and built up the African genome, supported and built up the genome of the plants that have substance affinities with the African genome, which is the establishment of the human genome in all individuals.

To support the healing cycle and homeostasis of the apparent multitude of organs and functions in the body, we have to re-visit a diet centered on the consumption of non-hybrid whole plant nourishments. This is health and healing. To speed recuperating or to reverse complex diseases, we ought to likewise re-visitation of utilizing natural alkaline non-hybrid plant herbs spices. The herbalist Dr. Sebi was urgent in restoring that antacid non-mixture plant nourishments had compound affinities with the body and upheld recuperating. His African Bio Mineral Balance procedure of recuperating depends on the reason that food that brings the corrosiveness level up in the body and that causes the overproduction of bodily fluid in the body is the foundation of sickness. Essentially, acidic and poison loaded nourishments persistently assault the body, cause a drawn-out incendiary response, and lead to chronic inflammation.

Intense irritation is a natural and health-supporting process used to battle infection and to fix actual harm done to the body. At the point when intense irritation isn't killed, the process at that point assaults healthy cells in different regions of the body and prompts the development of various forms of diseases. This tradeoff, the defensive mucous membrane that lines the organs and advances overabundance mucus creation, which thus bargains the soundness of organs. So, we start with eliminating these nourishments from the eating regimen, which incorporate meat, dairy, handled nourishments, and unnatural acidic hybrid plant food sources. A decent spot to begin is with this list of foods based on the alkaline nourishments suggested by Dr. Sebi.

ALKALINE PLANT FOODS AND HERBS SUPPORT THE ALKALINE BODY

The body capitulates to sickness when it is fermented. Acidifying the body bargains the mucous membrane that secures organs, which prompts the improvement of chronic illness. Despite the fact that the various areas of the body have different pH levels, we have to consume alkaline foods that keep up the 7.4 pH (a range somewhere in the range of 7.35 and 7.45) that the body maintains in the blood.

The term pH means "potential hydrogen" and is the capacity of molecules to pull in hydrogen particles or ions. The higher the pH the lower the measure of hydrogen is accessible. The lower the pH the higher the measure of hydrogen is accessible. The scale for pH goes from 0 to 14. The value 0 speaks to the most elevated acidic level, 7 are unbiased or neutral, and 14 represent the most elevated basic level.

Despite the fact that various pieces of the body have distinctive pH levels, the blood is a point of equilibrium and balance for homeostasis in the body. Homeostasis is the propensity toward a moderately steady balance between interdependent components. The body works constantly to keep up this steady harmony by conveying the nutrients that organs need to maintain health.

The blood needs to keep up a 7.4 pH before it can attempt to keep up homeostasis in the body. Metabolic acidosis happens when the blood's pH drops underneath this level, which can bring about stun and demise. It is critical to keep up this marginally soluble state in the blood since it lessens the measure of hydrogen in the blood. An excessive amount of hydrogen in the blood adds to the decrease of hemoglobin in red platelets, which hinders the best possible conveyance of oxygen and supplements to cells all through the body. This compromises the health of the organs and metabolic capacities.

The body has buffering frameworks set up that keep up the 7.4 PH. The buffering frameworks become overburdened when the body is continually taken care of acidic nourishments. The body will at that point take soluble material like calcium from bones and liquids all through the body to place into the blood to keep up its PH. This compromises the health of organs and their metabolic capacities and prompts the advancement of constant illnesses like osteoporosis, kidney sickness, heart infection, and liver sickness. Alkaline plant nourishments and spices keep up the blood's pH without the body compensate and compromise its health.

WATER

Water is regularly disregarded yet is fundamentally significant for supporting the solid articulation of the human genome. Products of the soil such as Fruits and vegetables contain a high grouping of water, yet individuals who consume a Western diet don't take enough foods grown from the ground. By and large, we ought to take one gallon of water a day, remembering water for food just like drinking water. The sure thing is drinking a gallon of water, and the body will dispose of what it needn't bother with. Springwater is the more secure water to drink. It contains characteristic minerals that cushion the water and ensure against destructive microbes. Drinking faucet water ought to be evaded. Faucet water contains added synthetic substances like chlorine to eliminate microscopic organisms and fluoride to ensure teeth, yet these synthetic substances are harmful to the body and subvert homeostasis.

ALKALINE MEDICINAL HERBS

The soluble development is running solid, because of crafted by the cultivator Dr. Sebi, who has initiated the alkaline development with his African Bio Mineral Balance. Numerous botanists utilize numerous different spices to switch infection. Dr. Sebi has been instrumental in recognizing the common soluble spices from these that best help the solid articulation of the African genome that is the establishment, all things considered. These spices are spicing whose compound piece hasn't been undermined through hybridization and hereditary alteration. The spices that have generally evolved in conditions of Africa or like Africa, under similar conditions as the African genome, have substance partiality with it. These spices help advance a climate of simplicity inside the body that upholds physical, mental, passionate, and profound security and revival in all individuals.

These spices fill in as an establishment for mending and switching infection. In spite of the fact that Dr. Sebi's rundown of spices that best help the African genome isn't comprehensive, these spices are separated from numerous other generally utilized spices that are crossover and acidic in nature. Despite the fact that these different spices do have some valuable properties, they additionally present mixes that don't have synthetic partiality with the body, cause issues with homeostasis and diminish the spice's adequacy. Spices like comfrey and even the mainstream Echinacea fall into this classification on account of their fragmented synthetic structure because of hybridization, hereditary, or organic control. I will address the alkaline spices Dr. Sebi uses to turn around sickness, which has been utilized for hundreds, if not thousands, of years in customary medication. I would likewise be neglectful to not distinguish a couple of spices that may not be essential for Dr. Sebi's rundown yet that are indigenous to territories that are like the climate of Africa, similar to the guinea hen weed of Jamaica.

HERBS AND THEIR PROPERTIES

(For educational purposes only, this information has not been evaluated by the Food and Drug Administration. This information is not intended to diagnose, treat, cure, or prevent any disease.) Some of the prescribes herbs and uses are listed below

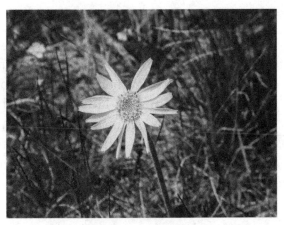

• ***Arnica*** (Arnica Montana, Radix Ptarmicae Montanae, arnica blossoms, mountain tobacco) is an incredibly calming and sterile spice. It is utilized fundamentally to treat outer injuries, and it soothes torment and advances tissue recovery. Arnica is utilized remotely as creams and packs to treat joint pain, injuries, wounds, and migraines. Arnica implantations are utilized for their sterile properties to clean injuries, abscesses, and bubbles. Dr. Sebi utilizes arnica as a component of his uterine wash compound. Inception: North America General business portion: Arnica is utilized basically as a skin cream.

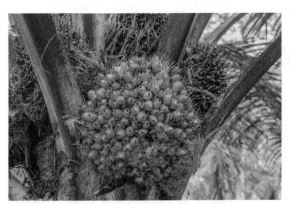

• ***Batana oil*** (Elaeis oleifera, American oil palm, palm oil) is produced using the piece of the product of the Elaeis oleifera tree. The oil is utilized basically for its unsaturated fats, supplements, and phytonutrients as a hair oil to reinforce hair, to advance its development, and as characteristic hair shading. It normally turns silver hair earthy colored. Root: Honduras, Central, and South America

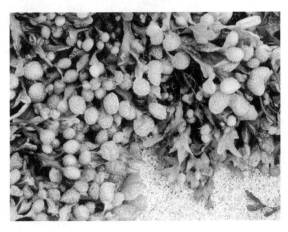

• ***Bladderwrack*** (Fucus vesiculosus, fucus) is utilized essentially on the grounds that it is a high wellspring of iodine. Bladderwrack has been utilized generally to treat an underactive and curiously large thyroid and to treat iodine insufficiency. Bladderwrack is likewise wealthy in calcium, magnesium, and potassium, and it contains other minor elements. Bladderwrack contains various phytonutrients, which are credited with its numerous medical advantages.

DR. SEBI'S HERBAL PRODUCTS

The herbalist Dr. Sebi has been instrumental in understanding the better alkaline herbs from the hybrid herbs that dominated the market. He was able to together herbal packages consisting of various herbs in specific doses to address varieties ailments. He has covered the properties of many of the herbs and uses them in his herbal packages. Also advise you to drink herbal teas than regular teas, like green tea, because they don't contain caffeine and contain a wide range of phytonutrients that support the immune system such as Alvaca, anise, chamomile, cloves, fennel, ginger, lemongrass, red raspberry, sea-moss tea.

CHAPTER 5

THE BENEFITS OF GOING PLANT-BASED

An ever-increasing number of individuals are getting mindful of the capacity of a whole food plant-based diet to help reduce and even fix numerous illnesses, for example, coronary illness, type 2 diabetes, joint pain, tumors, immune system sickness, kidney stones, incendiary inside infections and some more. Also, a plant-based eating routine is more affordable – particularly when you purchase a nearby natural product that is in season. So, we should look at a portion of the advantages of going plant-based.

1. *It Lowers Blood Pressure:* Plant-based nourishments tend to have a higher measure of potassium whose benefits, strikingly include diminishing pulse and mitigating pressure and tension. A few nourishments wealthy in potassium incorporate vegetables, nuts, seeds, entire grains and fruits. Meat, on the other hand, contains very little to no potassium.

2. *It Lowers Cholesterol:* Plants because they contain NO cholesterol – even the immersed sources like cacao and coconut. Driving a plant-based lifestyle will, subsequently, assist you to lower the degrees of cholesterol in your body prompting decreased dangers of heart disease. Checks Your Blood Sugar Levels Plant-based nourishments will in general have a ton of fiber. This hinders the ingestion of sugars into the circulation system just as keeps you feeling full for longer periods of time. It also assists balance out your blood cortisol levels thereby reducing stress.

3. *It helps prevent and fight Off Chronic Diseases*: In social orders where a larger part of individuals lead a plant-based lifestyle the rates of chronic diseases, for example, cancer, obesity, and diabetes are typically low. This diet has also been demonstrated to extend the lives of those already experiencing these constant sicknesses.

4. *It is good for Weight Loss*: Consuming entire plant-based nourishments makes it simpler to cut off abundance weight and keep up a more advantageous load without including calorie limitations. This is on the grounds that Weight misfortune naturally happens when you

consume more fiber, nutrients, vitamins, and minerals than you do animal fats and proteins.

PLANT-BASED DIET VERSUS VEGAN

It is very common for individuals to confuse a vegan lover diet with a plant-based diet or vice versa. Indeed, despite the fact that the two diets share likenesses, they are not actually the same. So, let's break it down real quick.

VEGAN

A veggie lover diet is one that contains no animal-based products. This incorporates meat, dairy, and eggs just as animal-derived products or ingredients, for example, nectar. Somebody who portrays themselves as a vegan carries over this point of view into their regular daily life. This means they don't utilize or advance the utilization of garments, shoes, embellishments, cleansers, and cosmetics that have been made utilizing material that originates from animals. Models here incorporate wool, beeswax, cowhide, gelatin, silk, and lanolin.

The inspiration for individuals to lead a veganism way of life regularly originates from a longing to hold fast and battle against animal abuse and poor moral treatment of creatures just as to advance basic entitlements.

PLANT-BASED DIET

An entire food plant-based eating routine on the other hand imparts a similitude to veganism as it additionally doesn't advance dietary utilization of creature-based items. This incorporates dairy, meat, and eggs. What's more is that dissimilar to the veggie lover diet, prepared nourishments, white flour, oils, and refined sugars are not part of the eating regimen. The thought here is to make an eating regimen out of negligibly prepared natural organic products, veggies, entire grains, nuts, seeds, and vegetables. Thus, there will be NO Oreo treats for you.

Entire food plant-based eating routine devotees are regularly determined by the medical advantages it brings. It is an eating routine that has next to no to do with confining calories or checking.

WHY YOU NEED TO CUT BACK ON PROCESSED AND ANIMAL-BASED PRODUCTS

You've presumably heard over and over that processed food is awful for the body. "Keep away from additives; evade processed foods"; notwithstanding, nobody actually truly gives you any genuine or strong data on why you ought to dodge them and why they are hazardous. So, let's break it down with the goal that you can completely comprehend why you ought to avoid these culprits.

THEY HAVE GIGANTIC ADDICTIVE PROPERTIES

As people, we truly have a solid propensity to be dependent on specific nourishments; however, the truth of the matter is that it's not altogether our issue. Essentially the entireties of the undesirable eat we enjoy, now and again, actuate our minds dopamine synapse. This causes the cerebrum to feel "great" yet just for a brief timeframe. This additionally makes a compulsion propensity; that is the reason somebody will consistently end up returning for another piece of candy – even in spite of the fact that they don't generally require it. You can evade this by eliminating that improvement through and through.

THEY ARE STACKED SUGAR AND HIGH FRUCTOSE CORN SYRUP

Processed and animal-based items are stacked with sugars and high fructose corn syrup which have near-zero healthy benefits. An ever-increasing number of studies are demonstrating what many individuals speculated up and down; that hereditarily altered nourishments cause gut irritation which thus makes it harder for the body to assimilate fundamental supplements. The drawback of your body neglecting to appropriately ingest basic supplements, from muscle misfortune and mind mist to fat addition, can't be pushed enough.

THEY ARE STACKED WITH REFINED SUGARS

Processed and animal-based foods are stacked with refined carbs. Indeed, it is a reality that your body needs carbs to give the energy to run body capacities. Nonetheless, refining carbs takes out the fundamental supplements; in the way that refining entire grains kill the entire grain segment. What you are left with subsequent to refining is what's alluded to as "unfilled" carbs. These can have a negative effect on your digestion by spiking your glucose and insulin levels.

THEY ARE STACKED WITH ARTIFICIAL INGREDIENTS

At the point when your body is burning-through artificial ingredients, it regards them as an unfamiliar object. They basically become an intruder. Your body isn't accustomed to perceiving things like sucralose or these counterfeit sugars. In this way, your body does what it does best. It triggers an insusceptible reaction that brings down your opposition making you powerless against illnesses. The concentration and energy spent by your body in ensuring your invulnerable framework could somehow or another is redirected somewhere else.

THEY CONTAIN SEGMENTS THAT CAUSE A HYPER REWARD SENSE IN YOUR BODY

This means they contain segments like monosodium glutamate (MSG), segments of high fructose corn syrup, and certain colors that can all things considered cut addictive properties. They invigorate your body to get compensation out of it. MSG, for example, is in a great deal of pre-bundled cakes. What this does is that it animates your taste buds to appreciate the taste. It gets mental just by the manner in which your mind speaks with your taste buds.

WHAT TO LOOK OUT FOR WHEN ADOPTING THIS LIFESTYLE

For a great many people hoping to go plant-based, protein is consistently a significant concern. There is this thought that is propagated by the traditional press upheld by enormous meat makers that protein is just found in meat. All things considered, that is simply false. Customary staples, for example, nuts, beans, oats, and earthy colored rice accompany a great deal of protein.

Frequently, supplements like calcium are promoted as originating from as if it was a creature-based source. Truly nourishments like kale, broccoli, and almonds contain bunches of calcium. Ask yourself this, in the event that calcium originates from meat, at that point where did the creature get it from? It's certainly from the greens they eat.

The significant worry for most plant-based eating routine supporters is typically nutrient B12. B12, for everybody, is normally found in sustained items, particularly grains and plant-based milk. In any case, those shouldn't be depended on to get enough of this significant nutrient. The most ideal alternative is to take a fluid or sublingual nutrient B12 supplement basically; just to ensure that there are no issues.

You can embrace a sound plant-based way of life by basing your eating regimen around cooked, what's more, crude nourishments loaded up with verdant and bright veggies. These will give your body the minerals, nutrients, and cancer prevention agents it needs.

CHAPTER 6

DR. SEBI FOOD LIST AND RECOMMENDATION

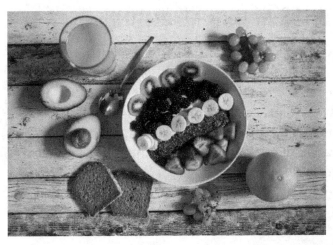

As purists will know Dr. Sebi would never recommend any foods that are not on his list of specifically recommended foods. These foods are known a Cell food. If you are looking to follow the alkaline food lifestyle diet you need to be aware of these recommended foods. This little guide is designed to help you choose these foods.

The Dr. Sebi food list is very specific; however, it surprisingly doesn't contain many very popular plant-derived/based foods that many people recognize as super whole foods. One surprising food that does not appear in this list is Garlic; Dr. Sebi regarded it to be dangerous and to be avoided at all costs. Dr. Sebi did not approve of hybrid foods, i.e. plant foods that are derived from unnatural cross-pollination of two or more different plants. These he regarded as genetically modified. The reasoning for this was he believed that hybrids altered the PH balance and the electrical composition, thus altering the genetic make-up to the detriment of the human body.

Here is a list of Dr. Sebi approved foods, that are recognized as suitable and safe for an alkaline diet for the human body. The Food lists are divided into categories, Vegetables, Fruits, Herbal teas, Grains, Seeds & Nuts, Oils, and Spices & Seasonings. Spices & Seasonings are further divided into Mild, Spicy, Salty, and Sweet.

VEGETABLES

Example of Vegetables Wild includes the following: Arugula, Avocado, Bell peppers, Cucumber Chayote (Mexican Squash), Dandelion, Greens, Garbanzo beans, Izote cactus flowers, cactus leaves Kale Lettuce except for iceberg Mushrooms and Shitake Nopales, Mexican Cactus Okra Olives Onions Sea Veg, -Wakame-Dulse-Arame-Hijiki-Nori Squash Tomatoes, -Cherry and Plumb only Tomatillo Turnip Greens Zucchini Watercress Purslane – Verdolaga.

THE BENEFITS OF VEGETABLES IN OUR NUTRITION

The Benefits of Vegetables is with the end goal that the absolute Most Essential Nutrients needed for the Day-to-day Functioning of the body is Found Nowhere Else, however in Fresh Vegetables! Because of the expanding demise rates and the sorts of persistent illnesses that have hit mankind, individuals have now begun grasping the advantages of vegetable sustenance. Remembering a decent extent of vegetables for our sustenance, if not a total vegetable eating routine, has its long just as transient advantages. Regardless of whether it is crude vegetables, cooked or made into juices, you will simply go gaga for these valuable greens for the marvels it can chip away at your wellbeing, notwithstanding the taste.

ADVANTAGES OF VEGETABLE DIET ARE ENDLESS

Why remember vegetables for your nourishment is a regularly posed inquiry by numerous who favor non-vegan over veggie lover diet. The way that vegetables are the prime wellspring of all generally a significant number of the nutrients and minerals of the solid working of the body makes them critical.

VEGETABLES ARE SUPER RICH IN NECESSARY NUTRIENTS

About 100% of the research state that vegetables frequently contain low fat yet being a rich wellspring of nutrients and minerals. On the off chance that you take a gander at vegetables at various tones, those going from green to orange give significant minerals like calcium, potassium, iron and furthermore a crowd of nutrients like C, K, An and so forth Another significant reality says that regarding half or a greater amount of the dietary fiber commitment as both solvent and insoluble is from vegetables, in this manner helping appropriate processing and admission of the food burned-through. Anyway, hard you may attempt, it can never so happen that your body can live without the assistance of these green marvels.

VEGETABLES HELP WARD OFF POTENTIAL HEALTH RISKS

On the off chance that you are searching for absolute avoidance and long-haul solution for any ongoing infections, like a malignant growth, cardiovascular sicknesses, joint inflammation, kidney inconveniences, and skin illnesses, better start remembering new vegetables for your nourishment. Aside from these, grasp and put to use the advantages of vegetables for better vision, cholesterol control, bettering the hemoglobin tally, and above all else keeping your body fit and solid.

VEGETABLES AID CONSIDERABLY IN WEIGHT LOSS

The advantages of eating vegetables are additionally exceptionally amazing to the stout. Considered as one of the prime common nourishments, it abandons referencing that vegetables are low in fat and calories yet is a decent fuel hotspot for the body. Additionally, with extensively low sodium levels, vegetables appreciate a spotless favorable position over prepared nourishments that not the slightest bit leaves a change to make you fat.

FRUITS

Oranges, peaches, pineapples, tangerines, or papayas are instances of leafy foods that are yellow/orange in shading. These nourishments bring a cell reinforcement, which diminishes cell harm; they likewise forestall coronary illness by lessening irritation. Another advantage of these hued nourishments is that they help keep bodily fluid layers and connective tissue sound.

RED/PURPLE/BLUE

Foods grown from the ground that are red, purple or blue in shading are wealthy in cell reinforcements that forestall blood clusters and secures against coronary illness. These nourishments likewise contain numerous enemies of maturing phytochemicals that keep the blood streaming. Instances of these leafy foods include: apples, blackberries, blueberries, cranberries, strawberries, beets, and so forth

Other red organic products, for example, tomatoes and watermelon, contain phytochemicals that lessen free revolutionaries in your body. These free revolutionaries can make harmful cells in the event that they come into contact with them so having less in your framework is something to be thankful for. Lycopene is extremely useful in forestalling prostate issues and diminishing the impacts of sun harm on the skin, it is additionally the explanation that these natural products have a red tone.

Consider making foods grown from the ground/vegetable plate of mixed greens to go with your next dinner. An extraordinary method to get whatever number of servings as could be allowed is to cause your plate of mixed greens to contain an assortment of shadings. Every last one of the shadings you drop into it will add explicit supplements to different parts of your body.

These are only a portion of the advantages that products of the soil bring into our day by day lives. These are likewise a few reasons why it is prescribed for us to allow 7-13 servings of products of the soil every single day to guarantee that we keep up a sound body. Our bodies are exceptionally mind-boggling frameworks of cells that require different nutrients and minerals with which to work appropriately, productively, and last more.

I have been supporting the advantages of a sound eating regimen in light of the fact that so a large number of us will in general disregard them. Numerous specialists concur that a solid eating regimen is a critical component in forestalling sickness. Also, two key components to a sound eating regimen are products of the soil. Despite the fact that we realize that this will generally be the situation, a large number of us actually don't get the necessary 7-13 servings of them daily. Indeed, even I, some of the time, miss a day or two and I'm viewed as a "wellbeing nut." That is the reason I take Juice Plus, it contains 17 natural products, vegetables, and grains in a couple of cases.

GRAIN

The principal advantage of entire grain nourishments is that they are processed more slowly than most nourishment. The slower processing of food positively affects our sugar and insulin levels, decreasing our danger of acquiring diabetes. Entire grain nourishments additionally help to forestall diabetes since they contain fiber. Studies have indicated that people who eat in excess of 5 grams of fiber consistently decline their danger of creating diabetes by 30%.

On top of forestalling diabetes, entire grain nourishments can likewise cut our danger of encountering a stroke or of creating malignancy. Studies have indicated that people who eat a lot of entire nourishments are at an essentially diminished danger of building up a feed and malignancy. Why? Since entire grains give our bodies a wide scope of supplements that help our bodies to ward off ailments and illness!

In the event that the diminished danger of diabetes, stroke, and malignant growth isn't sufficient to persuade you to change to entire grain nourishments, maybe its impacts on weight reduction will be. As referenced already, entire nourishments contain fiber. Fiber is a food source that really causes our stomachs to feel full quicker and more. Since we are full for more, we won't eat so a lot and will in this way lessen our everyday calorie admission and diminishing our measure of weight gain.

While eating entire nourishments for the duration of the day is significant, having them for breakfast is particularly advantageous. Entire grains contain starches, which furnish our bodies with energy. The additional energy that you get from an entire grain breakfast will give you a jolt of energy that can assist you with enduring a taxing day of work!

Like entire grains, nourishments, for example, natural products, vegetables, seeds, and nuts furnish our bodies with supplements that help to keep us and our bodies solid. For the most advantageous eating routine, make certain to eat in any event 3 servings of entire grains every day, with a mix of every one of different nourishments recorded.

SPICES

Spices are an extraordinary method to advance great health, particularly when consolidated effectively. Many give anti-inflammatory benefits; research shows that inflammation is at the root of numerous medical problems. Some give hostile to oxidant benefits, which help battle against free radicals, which lead to malignant growth. Here are twelve regular spices that ought to be staples in your diet.

- *Cumin*: A powerful anti-inflammatory, it is multiple times more powerful than nutrient C or E, and the early examination recommends it forestalls bosom, stomach, and colon malignancy. Cumin is found in curry (one of a few fixings) or can be utilized all alone. One tablespoon gives 20% of your everyday portion of iron, which assists with your energy level and safe framework. Early investigations show that it assists with memory.

- *Turmeric*: An amazing enemy of oxidant and mitigating, because of the Curcumin in it. It is best joined with dark pepper, as dark pepper contains piperine, which improves the assimilation of curcumin by 2,000 percent. In addition to the fact that it provides hostile to oxidant benefits, yet additionally invigorates the body's characteristic enemy of oxidant capacities. It brings down the danger of heart and cerebrum sickness, just as improves memory.

- **Cayenne Pepper**: This zest assists with awakening your digestion, assisting with weight reduction. It contains Capsaicin, which gives relief from discomfort (it is a functioning fixing in a few over-the-counter enemies of touchiness creams), battles prostate malignancy, stops ulcers, improved dissemination, standardizes pulse, and fortifies the heart. It likewise invigorates course and improves absorption. On the off chance that you are debilitated with seasonal influenza, it helps clear bodily fluid clog and assists with sore throat and hack.

- **Rosemary**: If you flame broil or sauté meat the cycle produces something many refer to as heterocyclic amines, which increment the chances of getting malignant growth. Marinating the meat in rosemary lessens the arrangement of heterocyclic amines by as much as 84%. It helps support fixation and mitigates pressure. It smells incredible as well.

- **Oregano**: Rich in nutrient K and a teaspoon gives as many enemies of oxidants as three cups of spinach. Nutrient K assists with blood thickening, fabricate solid bones, forestalls coronary illness, and works related to nutrient D (to the point that one doesn't work if the other is absent). Early examination proposes that oregano assists with forestalling this season's virus. It contains Thymol and Carvacrol, against bacterial operators that help battle contamination and have fourfold the counter oxidant levels that blueberries have. It helps ease feminine squeezing.

- **Cinnamon**: Eating a teaspoon daily of cinnamon lessens your danger for diabetes and coronary illness inside about a month and a half. It likewise assists with using glucose so you don't have the highs and lows that accompany eating sugars. It brings down cholesterol and helps keep your veins solid. It additionally mitigates acid reflux, sickness, fart, and lightens looseness of the bowels. It contains Glutathione, an enemy of oxidant that assists with dissemination.

- **Ginger**: There are various medical advantages to ginger, from helping settle a furious stomach to diminishing the irritation experienced from a decent exercise. It contains the compound Gingerol, which is accepted to be mitigating. The early exploration proposes that everyday use improves memory and core interest.

- **Nutmeg**: Nutmeg is valuable for acceptable oral cleanliness. It is brimming against bacterial mixes, for example, Macelignan, which decreases plaque and obliterates hole causing microorganisms. It is likewise a calming that smothers tumor development.

- **Garlic**: It is an enemy of contagious, an enemy of bacterial, and an enemy of viral specialist, and a few examinations show that it forestalls blood thickening.

- **Thyme**: The oil in Thyme is clean, an enemy of bacterial, and it helps battle MRSA contaminations, which are anti-microbial safe.

- **Sage**: This zest is brimming with rosmarinic corrosive, which is mitigating with a solid enemy of oxidant, which is known to bring down cholesterol and fatty oil levels. Studies propose it benefits memory, and is utilized with mellow Alzheimer's endures to help with that. In some cases, it assists with menopause.

- **Coriander**: This zest assists with bringing down glucose levels, and brings down cholesterol, decreasing the LDL cholesterol (the terrible kind) and expanding HDL cholesterol (the great kind). It is a characteristic anti-microbial that is successful against salmonella.

CHAPTER 7

DR SEBI'S CELL FOOD SUPPLEMENT

THE WHOLE FOOD SUPPLEMENT

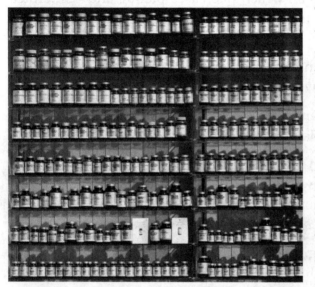

The effect of whole food supplements has been very favorably contrasted with artificial supplements such as multivitamins. The reason whole food supplements come out on top is simple: our body recognizes the ratios of nutrients in whole foods. It processes them far more easily than supplements consisting of isolated or fractionated nutrients. The body recognizes whole food supplements as nutritional and can metabolize and utilize them efficiently.

The best idea, say, experts, when it comes to determining your whole food supplements requirements is to decide on the readily available foods you can and will eat consistently and fill in the gaps. A general list of the most highly recommended vegetables regarding anti-aging and health benefits would include Kale, chard, spinach, broccoli, Brussels sprouts, cauliflower, red and green peppers, garlic, onions, sweet potatoes, tomatoes, green peas, asparagus, and carrots.

WHAT SUPPLEMENTS SHOULD YOU TAKE?

Whether you use vital nutrients as your barometer of what and how much to eat or as a guide in determining what whole food supplements you need, determining their presence or lack thereof is probably the best way to evaluate a diet. Below are some of the vital supplements most should consider alongside their diet, as recommended by Dr. Sebi.

- **Banju**: Dr. Sebi's Banju provides targeted nutrition and cleansing for the brain and nervous system. The tonic is rich in potassium phosphate to replenish minerals and antioxidants, reducing neurological inflammation.
  - Elderberry delivers a spectrum of flavonoids that protect and nourish the brain, enhancing neurological energy metabolism.
  - Blue Vervain delivers emotional and nervous restoration, reducing anxiety and relieving tension.
  - Burdock Root purifies and unifies the blood, increasing iron and oxygenation.
  - Valerian Root calms the nervous system: aiding peaceful and restful sleep, reducing irritability, and soothing pain.
  - The astringent Bugleweed supports detoxification and nourishes endocrine glands governing energy metabolism.

  The tonic enhances focus and cognitive functions, stabilizes emotions, balances the nervous system, and protects against oxidative stress.

- **Viento**: Dr. Sebi's Viento is energizing, cleansing, and revitalizing.
  - Enhancing circulation and oxygenation, the iron-rich capsules increase mental energy and physical stamina.
  - Chaparral supports lymphatic waste removal and expulsion of energy-draining heavy metals.
  - The potent antioxidant lignans reduce inflammatory damage, enhance immune defenses, and reduce addictive cravings.
  - Bladderwrack's nutritive iodides and cleansing bromides boost thyroid function, improving oxygen levels, energy regulation, and reducing appetite.
  - Valerian and Toad's Herb improve circulation, reduce stress, increase cellular oxygenation, and free up energy for vital immune functions.
  - Quassia Amara encourages the creation of oxygen-carrying red blood cells, enhancing cellular nutrition and energy production.

- o Invigorating herbs support your body's natural energy efficiency, boosting emotional stability, and mental clarity.

- **Testo**: Dr. Sebi's Testo boosts testosterone and enhances sexual virility. The potent herbs have helped thousands of men enhance sexual stamina, increase erectile strength, and reclaim sexual drive and desire.
  - o Sarsaparilla vine, an aphrodisiac native to Honduras, increases blood flow, helping the penis get engorged.
  - o Yohimbe, a West African sexual enhancer, contains testosterone-boosting alkaloids, enhancing vigor.
  - o Locust Bark's antioxidants and glycosides reduce inflammation and improve erectile blood flow.
  - o Capadulla, a Caribbean aphrodisiac, nourishes the whole urogenital system, preventing sexual decline.
  - o Irish Sea Moss is a remineralizing aphrodisiac, used since Roman times.
  - o Nopal supports the prostate, reducing inflammation and enhancing testosterone levels.
  - o Muira Puama stimulates libido and improves genital blood flow, naturally increasing penis sensation.

- **Iron Plus**: Dr. Sebi's Iron Plus is a nourishing and cleansing tonic that supports the blood and immune system. Antioxidants mitigate inflammation and help the immune system focus on rejuvenation.
  - o Elderberry's indigo-blue pigments mitigate free radical damage and reduce mucus.
  - o Blue Vervain & Chaparral, used traditionally by Native Americans, support digestive and respiratory functions.
  - o Hombre Grande and Quassia help purge parasites, mucus, and putrid waste from the bowel, while Palo Guaco reduces intestinal inflammation.

- Bugleweed's astringent aromatic bitters encourage detoxification and reduce endocrine inflammation.

- Cardo Santo, known as blessed thistle, regulates appetite, soothes indigestion, and helps regulate blood pressure.

- **Bio Ferro Tonic**: Dr. Sebi's Bio Ferro Tonic nourishes and cleanses the blood, supporting your immune system. Saturated with minerals and bioactive plant compounds, this liquid formulation provides deep cellular nutrition.

  Elderberry's rich indigo-blue flavonoids reduce inflammation.

  Chaparral used traditionally for arthritis helps remove toxins from the blood.

  Burdock's deep roots cleanse the blood, delivering oxygenating iron.

  Yellow Dock supports the circulatory system, reducing inflammation and blood pressure.

  Anti-inflammatory Cocolmeca promotes waste excretion and protects against cholesterol oxidation.

  Muicle helps cells respond to insulin, aiding blood sugar balance.

  Blue Vervain promotes restorative immune functions and reduces stress.

  Encino contains antioxidants targeting blood vessel inflammation.

- **Estro**: Dr. Sebi's Estro supports female reproductive health and hormonal balance. Targeted antioxidants and aphrodisiacs support libido and ease menstruation.

  - Hydrangea's flavonoids, saponins, and essential oils nourish the urogenital system while renowned aphrodisiac, Damiana, increases genital blood flow and sensitivity.

  - Anti-inflammatory Sarsaparilla reduces pain and enhances detoxification.

  - Irish Sea Moss balances the thyroid gland, while Muscle supports the production of new blood.

o Red Clover reduces hot flashes, soothes breast tenderness, and eases premenstrual or menopausal symptoms while relaxing.

o Blue Vervain reduces cramps.

o Muira Puama stimulates sexual desire and increases stamina.

o Abuta purifies the blood and stabilizes hormones, promoting emotional balance.

The potent herbs increase female sexual satisfaction, vaginal lubrication, and hormonal balance.

PART TWO
CHAPTER 1

DR. SEBI RECOMMENDATION FOR TREATMENT OF SOME ALIMENT

HIGH BLOOD PRESSURE

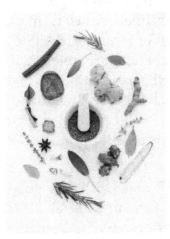

High blood pressure expands the danger of heart disease and stroke, two leading causes of Americans' death.

High blood pressure is also very common as tens of millions of adults in the world have high blood pressure, and many do not have it under control.

High blood pressure usually has no symptoms, so the only way to know if you have it is to get your blood pressure measured. This section of the book will help you on how you can manage your blood pressure and lower your risk.

DESCRIPTION

We can define blood pressure as a measure of the force that the circulating blood exerts on the main arteries' walls. The pressure wave sent along the arteries with each heartbeat is easily felt as the pulse—the heart contracts create the highest (systolic) pressure. The most minimal (diastolic) pressure is measured as the heart fills. Blood pressure is portrayed as a continuous variable, normally announced this way, with mean and standard deviation esteems. Relative danger esteems for the risk factor-disease relationship is likewise accessible for this configuration. The accepted unit for measuring blood pressure is mmHg, which may be applied to SBP, diastolic blood pressure (DBP), or alternative measurements such as mean arterial pressure and pulse pressure (PP).

Prospective researched studies have provided data on whether, over the long term, there appears to be an association between blood pressure and disease final-points. Therefore, an examination of the relationship strength for both DBP and SBP might be made. Information distributed from the Framingham study over the past 30 years has suggested that cardiovascular results don't get essentially from DBP (Kannel et al. 1969). While DBP may be a superior predictor of cardiovascular disease in those matured <45 years, SBP is a superior indicator of stroke and cardiovascular disease in those matured >60 years (Kannel et al. 1970, 1971).

Overall, the danger of cardiovascular events was greater in detached systolic hypertension than diastolic hypertension. For every standard deviation increment in mean SBP, the cardiovascular disease hazard expanded by 40–50%, while for DBP, the increment ratio was 30–35%. (This continued after changing of age and occurred in both men and women.) Combined systolic and diastolic hypertension conveyed hardly more serious risk than separated systolic hypertension (Kannel 1996).

Other prospective researched corroborate these results with evidence that, in both genders, the overall association between blood pressure and cardiovascular final-points is more grounded for SBP than DBP (Franklin et al. Comparative Quantification of Health Risks 1999, 2001; Lichtenstein et al. 1985; Miall 1982; Mitchell et al. 1997; Miura et al. 2001; Stamler et al. 1993; Sesso et al. 2000). A higher SBP was related to increased risk of IHD in a continuous and graded fashion in each DBP level. The risk with higher DBP within each SBP level increased, but the increases were not as steep or consistent (Stamler et al. 1993). SBP better-identified subjects who subsequently died from IHD than DBP. After all, SBP was a better predictor of outcome (Lichtenstein et al. 1985).

There are some data to suggest that PP (the difference between SBP and DBP) is a good predictor of cardiovascular risk (Abernethy et al. 1986; Black 1999b; Domanski et al. 1999; Frohlich 2000). However, it has not been consistently shown to be superior to SBP (Abernethy et al. 1986; Franklin 1999; Sesso et al. 2000; Franklin et al. 1999, 2001), and it was not a better predictor than SBP in the Asia-Pacific Cohort Studies Collaboration overview (APCSC 2003b); further, estimates of relative risk are available for SBP rather than PP. SBP was therefore used in preference to PP for these analyses.

HOW IS HIGH BLOOD PRESSURE DIAGNOSED?

Blood pressure is explained as part of a regular physical examined by the specialist or during most visits with a professional doctor. Individuals may have their blood pressure measured at a health center when they donate blood or are also involved in any medical screening.

If the outcome is high, the doctor will gather further information. For instance, the doctor will ask, if high blood pressure generally runs in the family tracts and what eating habits look like. It is considered essential to be careful of and let the doctor know salt intake in an individual's diet. Let your specialist know if salt is added during cooking or at the table if a lot of canned foods, frozen dinners, or highly salted foods such as peanuts or chips are eaten.

HOW IS BLOOD PRESSURE MEASURED?

The instruments called a blood pressure cuff are used in measuring blood pressure (The technical term for the tool is named sphygmomanometer.). Sphygmomanometers are put around the arm above the elbow, but different size arms require a different size. The cuff will produce an inaccurate measurement if it is too small or too large.

A tube attaches the cuff to an estimating gadget, and the cuff is siphoned loaded with air until the bloodstream in the main artery of the arm is shortly closed by the outside pressure.

A stethoscope is placed on the inward curve of the elbow over the artery so that the person examining the blood pressure can hear when the blood starts rising again through the route. The air is gradually released from the cuff, reducing stress on the arm and releasing the blood to flow once more.

The blood pressure readings: Systolic (known as the higher number) while diastolic (the lower number) is when pressure is most elevated and least during each heart cycle accordingly. Standard blood pressure is a systolic number of fewer than 120 and a diastolic number of under 80 readings. Likewise, blood pressure should be 119 over 79 or numbers less, not precisely those. It is quite possible to possess blood pressure that is too low. Low blood pressure has common symptoms like dizziness or fainting.

Note: If the blood pressure is observed between 120/80 and 139/89, this is known as prehypertension. This is not high blood pressure, but there is a likelihood of high blood pressure in the future. Prehypertension victims should take steps to forestall hypertension by receiving a healthy lifestyle. Also, normal blood pressure is less than 120/80. High blood pressure is reading more elevated than 139/89. A systolic reading of 140 to 159 and a diastolic of 90 to 99 is called Stage 1 Hypertension. A systolic reading of 160 or above and a diastolic reading of 100 or above is called Stage 2 Hypertension.

WHAT DO THE BLOOD PRESSURE NUMBERS MEAN?

A blood pressure perusing has a couple of numbers, for instance, 120/80. The primary, higher number, is the blood's weight in the vessels when the heart thumps and is known as the systolic pressure. The second, lower number, is blood pressure in the vessels when the heart is relaxed (diastolic) blood pressure. It is important for people to know and remember their blood pressure numbers! Be sure to ask what your blood pressure reading is each time you have it checked and record each reading.

WHY IS HIGH BLOOD PRESSURE UNSAFE?

High blood pressure makes the heart work more earnestly than ordinary to provide enough blood and oxygen to the body's organs and tissues. If high blood pressure isn't treated well; after some time, the heart tends to enlarge and weaken. A marginally enlarged heart may work just fine, but one that's fundamentally amplified struggles taking care of its responsibility and may ultimately fail. Likewise, high blood pressure increases the risk of heart attack, strokes, kidney damage, eye harm, congestive cardiovascular breakdown, and atherosclerosis.

WHERE CAN YOU GET YOUR BLOOD PRESSURE CHECKED?

Individuals can get their pulse checked at places in the community other than the specialist's office. Some of the spots where blood pressure can be checked are:

- Health fairs frequently have nurses or other medical personnel to check blood pressure

- Health facilities

- Fire department (do have medically trained workers to check pulse)

- Grocery store or medication store (will have a machine that can be used)

CAUTION: Automated machines may not be checked consistently for exactness or accuracy. Individuals ought not to rely on these machines alone for following their blood pressure measurements.

An individual can also screen their own blood pressure by taking it themselves. Simple-to-use monitors can be bought in drugstores and in the pharmacy section of large discount stores. Federal health care and private medical insurance will usually pay at least part of the cost of the blood pressure monitor. Ask the drug specialist about choices for paying for the monitor, and there may be resources in the community for helping to pay for the monitor.

Also distinguish places in your community that offer free or low-cost blood pressure screenings and monitors.

CAUSES AND SYMPTOMS OF HIGH BLOOD PRESSURE

WHAT CAUSES HIGH BLOOD PRESSURE?

Several conditions and practices add to high blood pressure. Some of the time high blood pressure is caused by another medical condition, such as kidney disease or lung disease. Below is the list of factors that leads to or cause high blood pressure.

- **Salt in the diet**: Most people devour more salt than their bodies required. A lot of salt intake can lead to an increment in blood pressure. Your everyday intake of salt ought not to be over 2300 mg or about 1 teaspoon of salt.

- **Being overweight or corpulent**: People who are overweight are bound to have high blood pressure

- **Lack of physical activity**: A minimal 30 minutes of moderate-vigorous active workout daily is suggested.

- **Heavy alcohol consumption**: If you consume alcoholic beverages, drink decently — for well-endowed men a limit of 2 drinks per day, and for women, a limit of 1 per day.

- **Race**: African Americans have high blood pressure since they are more averse to know about their blood pressure and are not being treated for it.

- **Age**: blood pressure tends to increase in line with age in many populaces, therefore aged individuals are bound to have high blood pressure.

- **Gender**: men have a higher risk of high blood pressure than their counterparts until age reached 55 when the risk becomes similar for both gender. At age 75 and more, ladies are more likely to exposure to high blood pressure.

- **Smoking**: Smoking influences blood vessels.

- **Diabetes and kidney disease**: People with such conditions are more at risk of a higher rate of high blood pressure.

- **Heredity**: people whose parents are inbound with high blood pressure are more likely to be infected than those whose parents are not.

WHAT ARE THE WARNING SIGNS/SYMPTOMS OF HIGH BLOOD PRESSURE?

Most of the time, there are no warning signs. A person can be calm and relaxed, and high blood pressure can still be present. A person can have hypertension for some years without knowing about it. High blood pressure is sometimes called "the silent killer." For these people, their blood pressure numbers are often their only warning.

However, some people with high blood pressure (especially if it is very high for a long time) can have one or more of the following:

- Tiredness
- Confusion
- Nausea or upset stomach
- Vision problems
- Nosebleeds
- Excessive sweating
- Skin that is flushed or red or skin that is pale or white
- Anxiety or nervousness
- Palpitations (strong, fast, or obviously irregular heartbeat)
- Ringing or buzzing in the ears
- Trouble achieving or maintaining an erection
- Headache
- Dizziness

The American Heart Association suggests that individuals have their blood pressure checked every two years. If the reading is high, however, they should have their blood pressure checked more often, as advised by their doctors.

REMEMBER: an individual can have hypertension and experience no symptoms.

PRECAUTIONS FOR AN HIGH BLOOD PRESSURE PATIENT

By living a healthy lifestyle, your blood pressure can be kept in a healthy range. Preventing high blood pressure, which is also known as hypertension, can lower your endangered risk for heart disease and stroke. Incorporate the following healthy living propensities:

EAT A HEALTHY DIET

Pick a healthy meal and snack options to help you avoid high blood pressure and its complications. Be certain to eat plenty of fresh fruits and vegetables. Talk with your medical services group about eating varieties of foods rich in potassium, fiber, and protein and lower in salt (sodium) and saturated fat. Mostly individual, making these healthy changes can help keep blood pressure low and secure against coronary illness and stroke.

KEEP YOURSELF AT A HEALTHY WEIGHT

Being overweight or corpulent increases the risk of hypertension. To decide whether your weight is in a healthy range, doctors often calculate your body mass index (BMI). On the off chance that you know your weight and tallness, you can compute your BMI at CDC's Assessing Your Weight site. Specialist sometimes also uses waist and hip measurements to assess body fat.

Talk with a professional medical care group about approaches to reach a healthy weight, including choosing healthy foods and getting regular physical activity.

DO NOT SMOKE

Smoking raises your pulse and puts you in more serious danger of cardiovascular failure and stroke. On the chance that you do smoke, quitting will lower your risk for heart disease. Your doctor can recommend approaches to help you quit.

LIMIT HOW MUCH ALCOHOL YOU DRINK

Do not drink an excessive amount of liquor, which can raise your blood pressure. Men should have no more than two alcoholic drinks per day, and women should have no more than one alcoholic drink per day.

GET ENOUGH SLEEP

Getting enough rest is important to your general wellbeing, and enough sleep is important in keeping your heart and blood vessels sound. Not getting enough sleep at a regular interval is linked to an increased risk of heart disease, high blood pressure, and stroke.

PREVENTIVE FOOD TREATMENT FOR THE REGULATION OF HIGH BLOOD PRESSURE

The following are necessary preventive recommendation/treatment by Dr. Sebi for patients having symptoms of High blood pressure or suffering from hypertension:

- Always ensure to drink a gallon of natural spring water daily.
- Must follow an alkaline plant-based diet recommended by Dr. Sebi which can be found in Book 2 which emphasizes Dr. Sebi's nutritional guide.
- Avoid table salt, only consume sea salt.
- Keep grains to a minimum, even alkaline grain
- Hypertension that is caused by another condition such as Thyroid or kidney issue must be addressed

BEST METHOD WHEN HEALING FROM CONTROLLING HIGH BLOOD PRESSURE

There are steps in a healing process that cannot be avoided if you want a positive result. These things will always remain the same regarding healing from any disease. They are as follows:

- **Cleanse the body**: The body must be cleaned on an Intra-Cellular Level through Detoxification in order to purify each cell in the body and remove Mucus. These can be achieved through Consuming Irish Moss, Spring Water, Herbs, Alkaline Fruit Smoothies as well as Tamarind and Green juice.

- **Detoxification**: It's a type of alternative medicine treatment that aims to rid the body of toxins which are substances that have accumulated in the body and have undesirable short-term or long-term effects on individual health.

- **Revitalize the body**: After fasting make sure that you consume herbs to nourish and replenish the body while strengthening the immune system. The body will then rebuild and rejuvenation will take place. Always consume lots of Sea Moss and Iron during revitalization.

According to Dr. Sebi in order to get rid of the hypertensive disease you have to clean the following; the skin, the liver, the gall bladder, the lymph glands, the kidneys, and the colon.

Above all only eat foods from Dr. Sebi's Nutritional Guide after completing your detox/cleanse.

DIFFERENT TYPES OF DETOX

Detox can be done in several ways. The common is through fasting. There are various fast including:

- Water Fast
- Liquid Fast
- Smoothie Fast
- Fruit Fast
- Raw Food Fast

HOW TO DO A DETOX

Depending on the fasting method that you choose, you want to focus on only consuming the drink(s) and/or foods that are specific to your fast for the specified amount of time. It is highly recommended that you also take cleansing herbs, which help to accelerate the healing process.

So, for example: If you are doing a water fast for 3days, you will only drink water while taking your cleansing herbs either in teas or capsule form. Nothing else should be consumed during those 3 days.

COMMON SYMPTOMS DURING DETOX

Here are the common symptoms you will likely experience during the process of detox:

- Hard Time Sleeping
- Feel Cold
- Cold &Flu Symptoms
- Tongue Discoloration
- Itching/Rash
- Aches & Pains
- Changes in Bowel Movements
- Low Energy
- Break Outs
- Expel Mucus
- Low Blood Pressure
- These are temporary and usually subside after the first week.

CLEANSING HERBS

Cleansing herbs to take while detoxing your body by Dr. Sebi Herb's treatment includes:

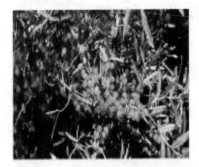

Sacred Bark: It causes muscle contractions in the intestines that help to move stool through the bowels while stimulating liver and pancreas secretion.

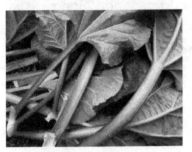

Rhubarb Root: Highly effective Laxative that helps improves tone & health of the digestive tract. Also cleanses heavy metals and kills harmful bacteria.

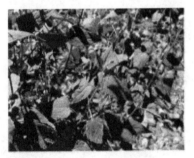

Brickellia: Stimulates pancreas secretions, reduces blood sugar level and motivates fat digestion in the gallbladder while improving stomach digestion.

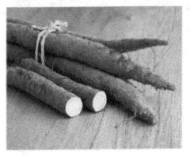

Burdock Root: Cleanse the liver and lymphatic system. Also helps to eliminate toxins through the skin and aids in the filtering of impurities through the bloodstream.

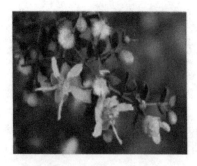

Chaparral: Cleanses lymphatic system and gallbladder. Also clears heavy metal from blood and helps to treat diabetes.

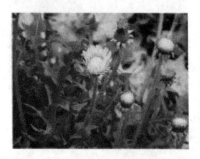

Dandelion: Cleanses kidney, gallbladder, and blood. Also dissolves kidney stones, provides relief from liver disorders, diabetes, urinary disorders, and is rich in calcium.

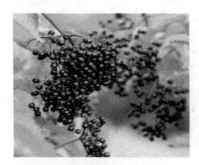

Elderberry: Removes mucus from the upper respiratory system and lungs. Increases urine flow and induces sweating.

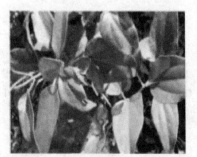

Guaco: Cleanses the blood and skin by promoting perspiration. Reduces inflammation, Increases urination and promotes a healthy respiratory system. Also high in iron strengthens the immune system and has potassium phosphate.

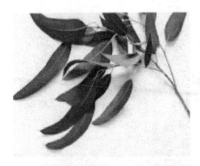

Eucalyptus: Can be used to help cleanse skin through steaming/sauna.

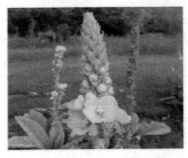

Mullein: Cleanse lungs, removes mucus from the small intestines, and activates lymph circulation in the chest and neck.

NOTE: It's a great benefit to cleanse at least once per year for 7 days if you are consuming an alkaline diet. If you are not eating alkaline foods from Dr. Sebi's nutrition guide, it is advised you cleanse/detox every 3 months. Also, keep in mind that consuming acidic foods will put the body at risk of relapsing for disease and if you have healed from a disease it will have your body at risk for relapsing depending on the disease.

CHAPTER2

LUPUS

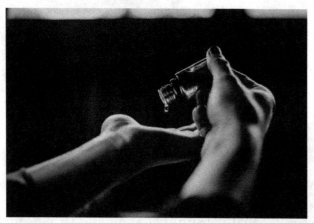

What is lupus disease? It's an inquiry that has baffled specialists and clinical scientists for quite decades, and there's still not a genuine, smart response to that question. Even though progressions have been made in lupus diagnosis and lupus treatment, the specific system that causes the sickness and the connections between hereditary, environmental, and hormonal elements or factors are unclear.

Lupus is classified as a chronic immune system infection. At the point when somebody has the infection, their insusceptible immune system goes haywire in a progression of flares (when lupus manifestations are available) and remissions (when an individual seems sound and doesn't encounter any side effects). Lupus sickness besets more than 1.5 million Americans and more than 5 million individuals around the world. Nine out of ten lupus patients are ladies and those in their childbearing years (ages 15-45) are the most susceptible even though the condition can influence individuals of all ages, both men and women.

DESCRIPTION

Lupus indications can keep going for quite a long time and can be hard to analyze as difficult to diagnose as they mimic the symptoms of several other diseases. In a typical, sound individual, the invulnerable system fends off and shields the body from foreign intruders. This incorporates microscopic organisms and viruses that the white blood cells perceive and wipe out by discharging protein antibodies that decimate the unfamiliar bodies. The immune system is simply the body's method of securing itself.

However, when an individual has lupus illness, the insusceptible immune system mistakes healthy tissues for unfamiliar intruders and assaults them with autoantibodies. Plainly, the body goes after itself and assaults its own cells and tissues. The final product is tissue damage, inflammation, pain, and even death in severe cases.

The skin, joints, and internal organs (the kidneys, lungs, heart, and brain) are most usually influenced; however, Lupus can affect all regions of the human body. The most well-known lupus manifestations in ladies and men incorporate fatigue, swollen joints, fever, discoid and butterfly rashes, and kidney nephritis, yet patients may likewise encounter a large group of different side effects. At the point when individuals notice the expression "lupus", they are generally alluding to foundational lupus erythematosus (SLE); however, the illness can take on a wide range of forms including discoid or skin Lupus, drug incited Lupus, and neonatal Lupus. Lupus treatment conveys with it a large group of side effects since it frequently includes the utilization of medications, for example, anti-inflammatory and corticosteroids aimed at reducing swelling.

TYPES OF LUPUS

There are five types of Lupus:

1. **SLE or Systemic lupus erythematosus**: This influences numerous parts of the body. The symptom of it can tend to be gentle, severe, and typically affects individuals within 15 to 45 years of age.

2. **Discoid Lupus**: This influences the skin. An individual with this sort of Lupus will have red and raised rashes that will happen for quite a period of days or weeks all at once.

3. **Subacute cutaneous lupus erythematosus**: This lupus type causes sores in the parts of the body that are usually under the sun. This doesn't cause scars.

4. **Drug-instigated Lupus**: Side impacts from prescriptions can cause this kind of Lupus. On most occasions, the lupus manifestations will disappear when the patient quit taking the medication that caused it.

5. **Neonatal Lupus**: This extraordinary kind of lupus influences babies that have SLE and different illnesses.

CLINICAL DIAGNOSIS OF LUPUS

The analytic cycle of Lupus is unpredictable, as the condition includes numerous influenced frameworks. A conclusion is made upon a patient's very own clinical history, actual evaluation, and demonstrative tests. These diagnostic tests include:

Hostile to DNA counteracting agent testing: This can give the most exact finding of the sickness (it was discovered to be exceptionally precise in one investigation); anyway, it demonstrates any connective tissue infection. What recognizes an SLE conclusion is the presence of other clinical signs of SLE. At the point when a patient has at least two clinical appearances of SLE and raised Anti-DNA antibodies, an analysis of foundational lupus erythematosus is affirmed.

Other research center pointers can be tried, and these include:

- **ESR** (erythrocyte sedimentation rate) is regularly raised: This test has been utilized for a long time to demonstrate aggravation is available inside the body. It is a basic and direct test.

- **Serum supplement levels**: These are done to quantify the action of specific proteins moving all through the blood, and demonstrate provocative cycles that are related to the invulnerable framework.

- **CBC** (complete platelet check) anomalies incorporate moderate to serious pallor, leukopenia and lymphocytopenia, and conceivable thrombocytopenia if there is Lupus present.

- **Urinalysis**: Shows gentle proteinuria, hematuria, and platelet projects during the compounding of the illness when the kidneys are included. Renal capacity tests incorporate serum creatinine, and blood urea nitrogen is likewise assessed.

- **Kidney biopsies**: May be performed to determine the extent of possible lesions. Clinical finding incorporates the taking of the patient's clinical history and an actual assessment and consideration of any of the above manifestations that are brought about by Lupus.

CAUSES OF LUPUS AND GENERAL SYMPTOMS OF LUPUS DISEASE

WHAT ARE THE CAUSES OF LUPUS DISEASES?

The reasons for Lupus are not actually known at this point. Nonetheless, it is accepted to be brought about by hereditary qualities, the climate, and hormones. The accompanying factors beneath are being considered by scientists to know whether these can likewise cause Lupus:

- Sunlight

- Stress

- Particular medicines

- Viruses and other infectious agents

An individual's insusceptible immune system with Lupus produces autoantibodies that assault joints and body organs as opposed to ensuring it. One of these autoantibodies is the Anti-Nuclear Antibody. The reasons for Lupus are still, to a great extent, obscure and aggravating the ambiguity is that every patient shows various indications.

GENERAL SYMPTOMS PRESENT IN LUPUS

Skin rashes are amazingly regular in individuals who are experiencing Lupus. A "butterfly" rash can commonly happen on the face, and it very well may be outwardly upsetting for the individual with Lupus. It can likewise be exacerbated from sun exposure. A vast larger part of individuals with Lupus likewise report having ulcerations in their mouths. Joint agony is one of the underlying markers of Lupus; a once in the past dynamic and solid individual having created joint torment and disquietude a potential pointer towards having Lupus.

Photosensitivity, where the skin can rankle from sun exposure, is likewise experienced IN individuals with Lupus. Fever and cerebral pains and THE announcing of headaches can be a continuous event because of having Lupus. Irritation of different organs, for example, the lungs can get hazardous if not treated. Alopecia (going bald) can be caused because of Lupus.

Individuals who have Lupus can infrequently encounter what is known as Raynaud's marvel — bloodstream confined to the fingers — causing deadness and cold; at that point, there is an abrupt surge of hot blood to the fingers causing extraordinary agony.

Insomnia can be a consequence of having Lupus, and furthermore many patients with lupus report having depression. Lupus can also cause issues, for example, inflamed kidneys, and subsequent impairment in kidney function, leading to the retaining of toxins in the body. This can cause the presence of blood in the pee, growth of the feet and lower legs, and dysuria. SLE can likewise cause the enlargement of glands.

BODY ORGANS THAT CAN BE AFFECTED

- Kidney: Nephritis will happen with no agony by any stretch of the imagination. At times, the lower legs of the patient will grow.

- Lungs: If the lungs are influenced, it will cause pleuritis that additionally causes the manifestations, for example, chest torment and breathing issues.

- Focal Nervous Symptom: If this is assaulted, this will cause the indications that happen in the head.

  o Veins: The individual with Lupus that assaults the veins will be prone to have vasculitis that influences the course of the blood.

  o Blood: If influenced, the individual can have iron deficiency leukopenia and thrombocytopenia, and strange blood coagulating.

  o Heart: The heart can have irritation whenever influenced by Lupus. This will cause chest torments and different indications of Lupus.

NOTE (Pregnant Women): Lupus indications in ladies will put her in danger on the off chance that she intends to get pregnant. She can have unsuccessful labor and untimely birth. A lady trying to get pregnant ought not to indicate Lupus or take meds for a half year before she tries to get pregnant.

NATURAL TREATMENT AND PREVENTION OF LUPUS DISEASE

If you are interested in preventing a lupus flare up one idea is not to smoke tobacco products. According to the U.S. National Library of Medicine, smokers were found to have significantly higher Lupus activity scores.

Another idea is to avoid too much sunlight. A good rule of thumb is to put sunblock on after 20-30 minutes of sun exposure. Next, avoid eating too much garlic. Garlic boosts the immune system, but with Lupus, a person has an overactive immune system and can increase the chance of a flare-up. Lastly, someone can take an omega 3 supplement.

Natural treatment of Lupus would be focused on the immune system part of the disease.

Homeopathy can help hugely treat immune system conditions; particularly because it focuses on the individual side effects every patient encounters. I will not suggest the Homeopathic treatment of Lupus as it is ideal to counsel a Homeopath while treating this condition with homeopathic medications. I will anyway make a recommendation on food treatment, spices, and diet in the treatment of Lupus.

DIETARY RECOMMENDATIONS FOR LUPUS PATIENTS

Eat asparagus, eggs, garlic and onions; these nourishments contain sulfur required for fix and modifying bone, ligament and connective tissue, and help in the retention of calcium. Incorporate earthy colored rice, fish, verdant green vegetables, non-acidic new natural products, oats, and entire grains. Eat new pineapple, as it contains bromelain for diminishing aggravation. Eat some type of fiber day by day.

Try not to burn-through milk, dairy, or red meat. Evade caffeine, organic citrus products, paprika, salt, tobacco, and sugar. Dodge nightshade vegetables, for example, peppers, brinjal, tomatoes, which may add to irritation. Keep away from horse feed.

SPICES

Ashwagandha tweaks and directs the resistant framework, which is significant in lupus patients. Lupus patients have a low degree of CD8 cells in contrast with solid people. CD8 cells are significant in regulating the overactive insusceptible framework, just like the case in immune system sicknesses. Ashwagandha assists with boosting CD8 cells.

Try not to utilize the accompanying: iron enhancements, as they may deteriorate irritation. Stay away from spices, for example, Echinacea, or any others that invigorate the resistant framework, as they can seriously exasperate Lupus. Tryptophan bothers System Lupus Erythematosus — along these lines SLE patients ought not to utilize supplemental Tryptophan.

HERB RECOMMENDATIONS FOR LUPUS

The top 3 herbs for autoimmune issues are ones use and help control flare-ups by Dr. Sebi. These are not typical immune-boosting herbs. In fact, using immune-boosting herbs can be a detriment. They can cause your immune system to go so far out of control it's literally eating you alive. No, we want herbs that are going to calm and regulate proper immune function. These herbs help bring things back to normal. There are specific herbs that will help you to protect certain organs and systems, but these ones work directly on your system.

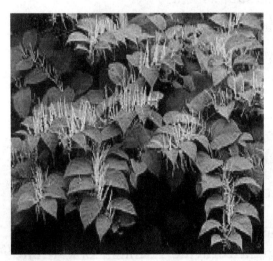

Japanese Knotweed: Not well known for immune issues, it really works. This herb is better known for being invasive and treating Lyme. This is one of 2 herbs that are making sensational headlines for being able to allow the body to completely rid itself of all Lyme bacteria and co-current infections. Knotweed does this by reducing inflammation and regulating the immune system. It allows the immune system to peak when fighting something, then to relax when the fight is over. For auto-immune issues, this herb calms the immune system down under normal conditions and allows it to work when an infection strikes.

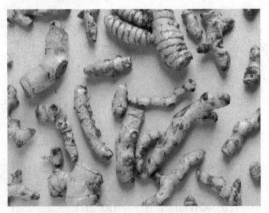

Turmeric: This super spice is here, too. This herb reduces inflammation by helping the adrenals produce anti-inflammatory hormones. It doesn't actually stop the inflammation, just works to keep it controlled. Turmeric also protects the body from attacks, including self-attacks. There are also now several studies that show turmeric can reduce the frequency and intensity of lupus attacks.

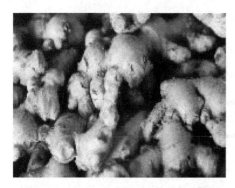

Ginger: It helps calm the digestive system and since there is more digestive system than the whole rest of the body combined, that's a good thing. Ginger also stimulates the body to reduce inflammation and supports the proper production of T-cells and other immune components. But, you need to be careful; too much for too long can have reverse effects.

GENERAL RECOMMENDATIONS

Get plenty of rest and regular moderate exercise. Avoid strong sunlight and use protection from the sun. Do not use birth control pills, as they can cause Lupus to flare up.

Excessive use of supplemental Estrogen by post-menopausal females increases their risk of developing Systemic Lupus Erythematosus (SLE).

"Disease can only exist in an environment that is acid…only consistent use of natural botanical remedies will effectively cleanse and detoxify a diseased body, reversing it to its intended alkaline state." Dr. Sebi.

CHAPTER 3

KIDNEY DISEASES

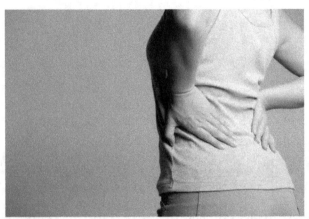

Our body system produces "nitrogenous" wastes when it metabolizes proteins and these are needed to be filtered from the blood. The kidneys are responsible for removing nitrogenous waste from the blood; these are the main functionality of such a powerful body organ. As channels, they remove the squanders and return clean filtered liquid to the body. The kidneys are generally comprised of miniature filters called glomeruli.

At the point when kidneys are sound and healthy, the arteries bring blood and wastes from the body into the kidneys, the glomeruli clean the blood, and the filters and additional liquid go out through the urine. Separated and purged blood leaves the kidneys and returns into the circulation system through the veins.

DESCRIPTION

To keep your body working appropriately, side-effects and overabundance fluid should be taken out consistently. To do this, it has two bean-molded kidneys each about the size of our clenched hand situated on one or the other side of your spine just underneath your rib cage.

The kidneys channel and re-visitation of the circulation system are around 190 liters of blood each day. So they produce up to 2 liters of pee that contain the byproducts your body needs to dispose of. The urine streams from your kidneys to your bladder. When your bladder is full, you get a desire to pee and the urine and the squanders it contains leave your body too.

Your kidneys additionally control electrolytes, keep up the corrosive base equilibrium, and keep your degrees of salt, potassium and phosphorus in line. By keeping up the salt and water balance, and creating the catalyst renin, they help manage your pulse. The kidneys likewise produce hormones that help make red platelets, just as a functioning type of vitamin D required for the wellbeing of your bones. As should be obvious, your kidneys are an essential piece of your body's cycles and have a ton of work to do.

The main substances excreted in the urine are:

- Metabolic waste products such as urea and creatinine from the chemical processes (such as digestion) that keep your body functioning
- Electrolytes- inorganic compounds (including sodium, potassium, calcium, chloride and bicarbonate) that your body uses to control its fluid content
- Water.

HOW KIDNEYS ARE DAMAGED

There are two broad types of damage to your kidneys:

- acute kidney injury, and
- chronic kidney disease

Acute kidney injury, also known as *acute renal failure* (ARF), is a sudden loss of kidney function. There are many ways in which this can happen. ARF can occur following:

- A sudden reduction in the flow of blood to the kidneys due to a traumatic injury with severe loss of blood
- Damage to the kidneys due to shock from a severe infection
- Damage from toxins or certain drugs
- Obstruction of the flow of urine
- Complications during pregnancy

Runners who don't drink enough fluids when competing in long-distance endurance events can suffer a sudden breakdown of muscle tissue. The breakdown releases myoglobin, a protein found in muscle tissue that only appears in the bloodstream after muscles are injured; this protein can damage the kidneys severely and result in ARF.

KIDNEY DISEASE

When the kidneys are healthy, the microfilters in your kidneys keep protein inside your body. High blood glucose and high blood pressure damage the kidneys' filters. When this happens, protein leaks out of the kidneys and into the urine. Damaged kidneys aren't able to filter out wastes and extra fluid from the blood instead of leaving the body in urine. Kidney damage doesn't show symptoms early on. An early sign of kidney damage is when your kidneys leak small amounts of a protein called albumin into the urine, and this is why the annual urine test is recommended. As the kidneys become more damaged, they leak more and more protein.

Kidney damage from diabetes happens slowly, and you may not feel sick for many years. You won't feel sick even when your kidneys do only half the job of normal kidneys! You may not even feel any signs of kidney failure until your kidneys have almost stopped working. This is why it's so important to get your urine and blood checked every year. That way your doctor can tell you how well your kidneys are working. Signs of failure are: feeling sick to your stomach and tired all the time. Your hands and feet may swell from extra fluid in your body. Kidney stones are pieces of hard solid matter made in the kidneys from minerals in the urine. They are formed when there is too much of a particular substance (such as calcium) in your urine. They can vary in size from as tiny as a grain of sand to as big as a pearl or (rarely) a golf ball. Kidney stones usually go down the urinary tract and pass out when you urinate. Indeed, many stones are formed and passed without causing symptoms. But if the stones grow large enough (at least 3mm) they can block the urethra. This causes pain, beginning in the lower back and radiating to the groin. Other symptoms include nausea, vomiting, fever, blood in the urine, and painful urination.

One of the major causes of the formation of stones is dehydration due to a low intake of fluids. The risk of forming kidney stones is increased when you eat lots of animal protein, salt, refined sugars, fructose, and high fructose corn syrup. Drinking grapefruit and apple juice also increases the risk.

Developing kidney stones can run in the family. The best way to prevent stones from developing is to drink enough fluids that you produce more than two liters of urine every day and adhere to a low-sugar, low-salt diet that contains minimal animal protein. You should also avoid drinking colas.

CHRONIC KIDNEY DISEASE

Kidney damage that lasts longer than three months is known as *chronic kidney disease* (CKD). It is particularly dangerous because you may not have any symptoms until considerable (often irreparable) damage has been done.

The two most common causes of CKD are:

1. Diabetes (both types 1 and 2), and

2. High blood pressure

Other causes of CKD include chronic viral illnesses (such as HIV/AIDS and hepatitis B and C), urinary tract infections within the kidneys themselves, inflammation following a strep infection, congenital defects, toxins, some medical drugs, and the use of recreational drugs that are injected. You can also damage your kidneys by eating too much animal protein and not drinking enough water.

Your kidneys are made up of millions of extremely small filtration units that purify your blood and send the waste products out into the urine. These tiny filtration units can be damaged by high glucose levels (diabetes) and high blood pressure (hypertension).

Unused glucose in your bloodstream is filtered by your kidneys and then normally reabsorbed back into the bloodstream. However, there is a limit to the rate at which the kidneys can filter and return glucose. When this limit is exceeded — as it can be if you don't get your diabetes under control — your kidneys become stressed from over-work and the glucose starts to spill into the urine.

Your kidneys are particularly sensitive to high blood pressure. At the same time, they play an important role in the regulation of blood pressure and if they have been damaged, they can lose some of their ability to keep blood pressure down.

The problem is circular — high blood pressure damages the kidneys and damage to the kidneys can contribute to high blood pressure.

BEATING KIDNEY DISEASE

In the early stages of the disease, there are usually no symptoms. But as things get worse, changes in bathroom habits — having to go more or less often — can signal a problem. You may also feel tired, have muscle cramps, lose your appetite, and have swollen hands or feet, and dry, itchy skin.

The only fix is to regulate your blood pressure, using medication prescribed by your doctor and beat the effects of diabetes by following a low-sugar, low-fat, low-salt, and high-fiber diet and avoiding eggs and dairy products.

Getting both your blood pressure and blood glucose levels under control is imperative because once your kidneys stop working your body begins filling up with wastes, fluids, and toxins. With your kidneys out of action, the only way to get rid of these is to go on dialysis — using a machine that acts as an artificial kidney, cleaning your blood — a very inconvenient, extremely messy, and highly uncomfortable procedure.

If you allow damage to your kidneys to develop, you will end up needing kidney dialysis at least three times a week. In the end, you will probably need a kidney transplant.

Above all else, drink plenty of water. Check when you go to the toilet: is your urine clear to light yellow? It should be — if you are drinking enough liquids.

WHAT HAPPENS IF SOMEONE GET DIABETIC KIDNEY DISEASE?

One way to treat diabetic kidney disease is with dialysis. Dialysis is a treatment that filters your blood the way your kidneys used to do. There are two types of dialysis are available. You and your doctor will decide what type will work best for you.

Hemodialysis.

In hemodialysis, your blood is taken through a tube from your arm to a dialysis machine that filters out the waste products and extra fluid. The clean blood flows back to your arm.

Peritoneal dialysis.

In peritoneal dialysis, your abdomen is filled with a special fluid. The fluid absorbs waste products and the extra water from your blood. The dialysis fluid is then drained from your belly and discarded.

Another way to treat diabetes kidney failure is to have a kidney transplant. The kidney can be from a close family member, perhaps from a friend, or even someone you do not know. It's all a matter of finding a good tissue match that your body will accept. Many people are waiting for a new kidney, so you may be on dialysis for quite a while. The functioning of your kidneys can deteriorate for a variety of reasons.

Other Kidney diseases include:

- Hypertension: Also a leading cause of kidney disease, as well as heart attacks and strokes

- Glomerulonephritis: Inflammation of the kidney's tiny filtering units

- Polycystic kidney disease: The most common inherited kidney disease

- Urinary tract infections: Most often affect the bladder but can spread to the kidneys

- Congenital diseases: That involve some problem in the urinary tract

- Pain relievers: Long-term use of over-the-counter pain relievers

- Recreational drugs: Such as crack and heroin

- Toxins: Such as obtained from pesticides

Uncontrolled high blood glucose and high blood pressure are, by far, the most common reasons for the deterioration in kidney function. There are plenty of things you can do to prevent the destruction of your kidneys.

HERBAL MEDICINE TO TREAT KIDNEY NATURALLY

The doctor may have told you that your kidney is a problem. You may still be afraid that you may have Kidney Failure. Whatever your situation, knowing what the most effective herbs for kidney symptoms could be found in herbal leaves called "Sambong Leaves."

SAMBONG LEAVES: THE MOST POWERFUL HERBS IN KIDNEY DISEASE

The sambong leaves are very effective herbs for kidney disease because it is a popular diuretic and helps to improve the body's ability to maintain water. Sambong herb was also recommended by Dr. Sebi during kidney treatment The tea made from the sage is when consumed helps the body pierce much to remove excess water and salt. Studies show that high saltiness in the body is one of the main causes of high blood pressure.

The sage is the only herbal medicine approved by the Philippine National Kidney and Transplant Institute as an herbal medicine herb that has the ability to slow down or prevent renal failure. Thus, this Philippine National Kidney will recommend the use of sage tea "sambong leaves" or any other forms of kidney Dysfunction. Interferes have shown good effects that help prevent the patient from possible dialysis or a kidney transplant.

The "sambong leaves" sage is also known as kidney stones. The Department of Health of the Philippines recommends drinking health supplements made in the "sambong leaves" sage as a diuretic and for digestion of kidney stones to treat kidney failure.

PREPARATION OF HERBAL MEDICINE FOR KIDNEY DISEASE

Here are the steps to make "sambong leaves" sage tea:

1. Take a leaf of "sambong leaves" sage and cut them into small pieces.

2. Wash them with clean water

3. Boil 50 grams of sage leaves in one liter of water

4. Let it be within 10 minutes.

5. Drink hot or cold depending on personal preferences

PREVENT KIDNEY DISEASE

According to experts, the most effective way to prevent kidney damage is not to take medicines for kidney, but to avoid having kidney failure.

Here are the golden rules to prevent kidney disease:

- Stay fit and active
- Control blood sugar
- Eating healthy and maintaining proper weight
- Drink plenty of water
- Do not smoke
- Avoid unnecessary drugs, supplements, and toxins.

CHAPTER 4

HERPES

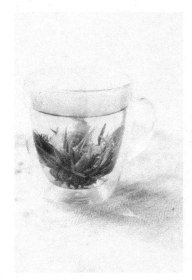

The complexity of the virus that causes herpes often leads people to ask: What is herpes? In actuality, there are two viruses that cause the condition to develop in men and women: simplex 1, or HSV-1, and simplex 2, or HSV-2. These two strains are very similar, and yet very different from one another. When broadly asked what is herpes, one can answer by saying that it is a virus that results in reoccurring appearances of "outbreaks," which are clusters of small blisters and ulcers similar to cold sores. The virus is not always active and may remain dormant in a person for months or even years. There are no known cures for it, and there are numerous medical and natural treatments available to help remedy the often painful physical effects of the virus. There is an oral variety as well as the more feared genital case.

DESCRIPTION

WHAT IS GENITAL HERPES?

It is a sexually transmitted disease affecting the genitals and anal areas of both men and women. This form of herpes—usually HSV-2—is far less common than the oral form of the virus, HSV-1, but the sores' progression is generally the same, as is the means of transmission. The skin to skin contact of a person who is currently suffering from an outbreak to another person during sexual intercourse is the leading cause of transmitting the disease.

Unlike HSV-1, the spread of the HSV-2 virus usually occurs later in life, and most people who have the second form of the virus don't get it until they reach adolescence or adulthood. Studies regarding the HSV-2 virus have indicated that about 20% of the American population is afflicted with the virus.

WHAT IS ORAL HERPES?

This form of the virus is commonly visible to the general public. It is the formation of cold sores on one's lips, mouth, or surrounding areas. It is often contracted by children at a young age, although it can be contracted during adulthood as well. What is oral herpes spread by? Skin to skin contact with an individual amid an outbreak causes the spreading, although not all outbreaks are visible. In rare cases, the HSV-1 virus can contaminate the carrier's eye, which results in the development of ocular herpes.

Studies have reported that almost 80% of Americans have the HSV-1 virus within their body. However, the development of immunities to the virus in the body often suppresses sores' formations as people age. By the time most people with the virus reach adulthood, the HSV-1 is usually lying dormant within the body.

CAUSES OF HERPES DISEASES

A herpes outbreak is caused by the simplex virus activation in the spinal cord nerves. Generally, the Herpes simplex virus remains dormant in the sensory nerve cells and is triggered by varying biological influences. During its onset, Herpes travels to the skin leading to an outbreak characterized by blisters or sores. In some instances, herpes may only emerge as painless irritated and cracking skin. The previous blisters or sores, however, are generally excruciating and difficult to deal with.

Many researchers have found little evidence that affiliate stress or individual diets as a factor in herpes outbreaks. Although the evidence is lacking, it doesn't mean that it doesn't exist. The usual activating causes are afflictions or traumas that affect the skin or mucosal membranes of the genitals. Ultimately, though, very little is known about the activation itself.

What is particular with herpes outbreaks of simplex type 2 is that they will occur between four and six times per year if left untreated. The actual shedding of the virus can happen up to twenty percent of days without the appearance of a breakout or symptoms. The general method of suppression is therapy using oral prescriptions that can drastically reduce herpes outbreaks.

Both herpes virus simplex 1 and herpes virus simplex 2 are microscopically identical and share about half of their DNA structures. All herpes infects the mucosal areas of the body — generally the lips and genital areas — and remain with the central nervous system during other times.

PREVENTION

The first thing that you want to know is probably what causes an outbreak in the first place. There is no single cause of a herpes outbreak. It is actually a combination of many factors. Poor health is definitely one of them. Your immune system should be in tip-top shape if you want to avoid a herpes outbreak from happening. Try to eat healthy foods as much as possible. You should also exercise regularly and make sure that you are getting enough rest.

Stress is another thing that is known to cause a herpes outbreak. People who want to know how to prevent herpes would probably be surprised by the condition's connection with stress. Stress can also affect the immune system negatively. With a lowered immunity, our body is open to all kinds of infections, including a herpes outbreak. So try to deal with the things that give you stress daily.

GENERAL SYMPTOMS

Even if someone is infected with genital herpes, but not having the symptoms of herpes, another person can still get infected. Someone infected with herpes may not even know they have it, as the disease can lie dormant for years, but eventually, something will set the virus off for the outbreak to start. Although there is no cure for genital herpes, you can get treatment for symptoms that you will eventually get.

Once you start to experience the disease symptoms, they generally appear between four to seven days once you have been infected with the disease. The first time you are infected with the disease is the primary infection, which tends to be the worst infection. Further infections later are called recurrent infections, and these tend to be not as severe.

SYMPTOMS OF THE PRIMARY INFECTION CAN INCLUDE THE FOLLOWING

- Vaginal discharge in women.
- Ulcers, blisters on the cervix in women.
- Excruciating sores or blisters around your buttocks, anal passage, genitalia.
- Pain when you are passing urine.
- A very high temperature, fever, and generally feeling unwell with bad aches and pains.

All these symptoms can be present for up to at least twenty days, but eventually, will all disappear, including the sores, blisters which will heal completely.

SYMPTOMS OF RECURRENT INFECTION

Once the primary infection has been treated, it will lie dormant in your nerves and eventually will trigger the recurrent infection, which will include:

- Itching and tingling feeling around the genitals, down the leg sometimes, before the blisters come back. This is usually the first indication that the recurrent infection has started.
- Excruciating sores around the genitals, rectum, and thighs, and bottom.
- Painful blisters or sores in the cervix of women.

These symptoms are not as severe as the first infection because they have learned to fight the infection by producing antibodies to fight it. Generally, the recurrent infection can last up to ten days, and you won't have a severe temperature or feeling unwell.

TREATMENT

The treatments for both forms of the disease are almost identical. These treatments include a variety of prescription medications, as well as natural home remedies. Because prescription medications often result in varying degrees of unwanted side effects, more people have been turning to more natural methods to ease the symptoms of the virus. Studies have shown that vitamin C, lysine, and Dr. Sebi are all effective ways to treat both forms of the herpes virus.

The symptoms of herpes can be healed or prevented by using natural herbs. Some of the herbal treatments for herpes are essential oils, tinctures, and herbal teas. The herbal treatments can be used topically or orally and you don't have to worry about any side effects. For decades now, these herbal treatments have been used by many people. Read on to find out what herbs are best used to treat herpes.

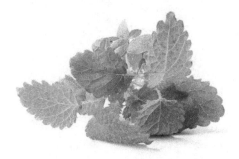

Melissa or lemon balm is quite expensive but you can easily find them in the market. To avoid oral herpes, add a few drops of the essential oil to the day cream you're using. Lemon balm is also available in tea form and you can drink it every day for more effective results. You can create your own tea by chopping lemon balm leaves. Use two teaspoons of lemon balm for a cup of water and boil it; brew it for another ten minutes.

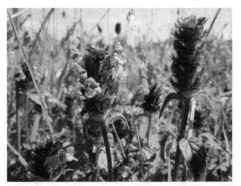

Prunella vulgaris is another herbal treatment that you can use. This herb is also called 'heal-all' or 'self-heal'. By mixing this herb with olive leaf extracts, lysine, and vitamin C. This mixture can suppress the outbreak of herpes.

You can also use Siberian ginseng or Eleutherococcus to treat type 2 herpes virus. You can't use this herb for treating type 1 HSV though. Oftentimes, herpes and cold sores are due to stress. Ginseng helps in dealing with mental and physical stress due to exposure to viruses, physical exhaustion, pollution, noise, chemicals, and other things. Ginseng can also stimulate the immune system thereby preventing outbreaks. However, individuals suffering from apnea, narcolepsy, and high blood pressure should not use Siberian ginseng. Breastfeeding mothers and pregnant women are also not allowed to use such herbs.

Some herbalists say that herbs are much more useful when taken in liquid form. Any kind of tea can ease the HSP type 1 symptoms since the flavonoids and polyphenols boost the immune system. Some studies also show that HSV type 2 can also be suppressed by drinking tea regularly. Once the immune system is stimulated against viruses and bacteria, it will inhibit the occurrence of the two types of HSVs.

White and green teas are quite effective and you must take them regularly. Some individuals say that by applying the tea bags or brewed tea to the infected area, the healing process is faster which can only take 4 days. Tea tincture is also good for healing herpes. It would be best to choose teas without caffeine for the best results.

PART THREE

FOOD RECIPES

INTRODUCTION TO FOOD RECIPES

"Everyone should be his own physician. We ought to assist and not force nature. Eat with moderation what agrees with your constitution. Nothing is excellent for the body but what we can process and digest. What medicine can produce digestion? Exercise. What will recruit strength? Sleep. What will alleviate incurable ills? Patience."

– *Voltaire-*

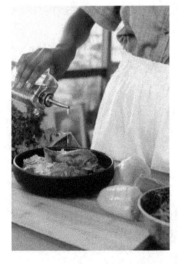

Everyone is baffled about what is right to eat nowadays. Several diets range from eating only plants to eating a diet primarily of animal foods—vegan, vegetarian, Mediterranean, Paleo, grain-free, raw food diet, and everything in between. Proponents of each diet proclaim that they know the ticket to health, justifying their points with well-documented research and case studies. For many, creating nourishing meals has become confusing and stressful rather than a joyous process.

Dr. Sebi food in particular; however, it surprisingly doesn't contain many very popular plant-derived/based foods that many people recognize as super whole foods. His food recommendations are specific foods recommended for sound health proven from research and studies. These foods are known as Cell food and are categorized into different sections. The Food which are divided under categories of Vegetables, Fruits, Herbal teas, Grains, Seeds & Nuts, Oils and Spices & Seasonings, and food are sub-divided into Mild, Spicy, Salty and Sweet.

In the next chapter of the book, we will be discussing the recipes of a few selected food out of the list of approved food based on Dr. Sebi's nutritional guide.

SALAD RECIPES

INTRODUCTION

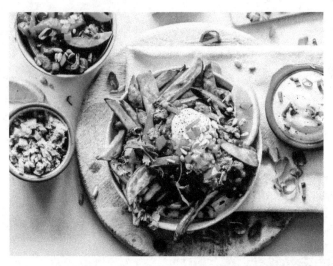

When it's burning up outside, the last thing you (probably) want is a big bowl of hot soup or a heavy pasta dish. No, a pleasant plate of mixed greens is something that certainly sounds a great deal more invigorating. It's quick and easy to make, there are million-and-one options to choose from and, it's also a healthy meal that will help keep you cool and satisfied.

Salad can be pressed loaded with effective supplements, contingent upon the assortment of vegetables you put in them. Additionally, the measure of calories in your salad can fluctuate broadly on account of the sort of cheese, dressing, nuts and protein added to it. A scientific study revealed that regular salad eaters have higher nutrient levels in their bloodstreams than non-salad eaters. They tend to have high levels of vitamin C, folic acid, alpha and beta carotene, lycopene and vitamin E through the presence of the vegetables in salads.

SALAD AND NUTRIENTS

Salads can be an excellent way to get your essential vitamins and minerals. Salads also supply fiber. However, not all salads are healthy or nutritious. It depends on what is in the salad. It is OK to add small amounts of dressing and toppings, however, if you overdo it with high-fat add-ins, your salad may cause you to exceed your daily calorie needs and contribute to weight gain.

Prepare salads with colorful vegetables. If you have plenty of fresh vegetables in the salad, you will get healthy, disease-fighting nutrients.

DR. SEBI DIFFERENT DRESSING OF THE FOOD SALAD

There is a different type of alkaline salad dressings in which Dr. Sebi recommends any of the three; Mango Papaya Seed, Cucumber Dill, and Red Ginger. Be mindful of the extra items you add to your vegetable salads, which may be high in saturated fat or sodium. Here are different recipes for the dressing of other type of salad:

You want to include some fat in your salad. Mixing vinegar with olive oil or other vegetable oil is a good base for homemade dressings. You can also add nuts and avocado to include healthy fats. This will help your body make most of the fat-soluble vitamins (A, D, E, and K).

Use salad dressing or added fats in moderation. Large amounts of prepared salad dressing or toppings such as cheese, dried fruits, and croutons can turn a healthy salad into a very high-calorie meal.

Chunks of cheese, croutons, bacon bits, nuts, and seeds can increase sodium, fat, and calories in a salad. Try to choose only one or two of these items to add to your colorful veggies.

At the salad bar, avoid add-ons such as coleslaw, potato salad, and creamy fruit salads, increasing calories and fat.

Try to use darker lettuce. Light green Iceberg has fiber but not as many nutrients as dark greens such as romaine, kale, or spinach.

Add variety to your salad with high-fiber items such as legumes (beans), raw vegetables, fresh and dried fruit.

Include a protein in your salads to help make them a filling meal, for example, beans, grilled chicken breast, canned salmon, or hard-boiled eggs.

CUCUMBER TOMATO SALAD

Cucumber Tomato Salad is a super simple healthy salad that packs a punch of flavor. You'll love the delicious lemon dill dressing!

Ingredients

2 English cucumbers, diced
1-pint cherry tomatoes, quartered
1 red onion, diced
2 tablespoons extra virgin olive oil
2 tablespoons lemon juice
1 tablespoon apple cider vinegar

1 teaspoon granulated sugar or honey
1 teaspoon salt
1/2 teaspoon black pepper
2 tablespoons fresh dill, minced

Instructions

1. Dice your cucumbers into sizeable pieces

2. Cut your cherry tomatoes into half if small or in quarter

3. Give your red onion a quick dice.

4. In a large bowl, pour all your toss cucumber, tomatoes, and onion together.

5. In a small bowl, whisk together olive oil, lemon juice, vinegar, sugar, salt, pepper, and dill.

6. Pour over cucumbers and toss to combine.

7. Cover and refrigerate at least 1 hour before serving.

AVOCADO SALAD

This is an easy and super healthy100% vegan salad recipe under 10 min; no oils or salt added could be great for dieting and health reasons. Super nutritious. It can be dressed with any choice of salads.

Ingredients

2 Avocados

A little amount of chop Pineapples

1-pint Tomatoes

1 Red onion

1cup Corn

2teaspoon Thyme

Parsley

2 Garlic

½ Sprin onion

1/2 teaspoon black pepper

3 bell pepper

Instructions

1. Dice your Avocados and pineapple into sizeable pieces

2. Cut your tomatoes and bell pepper into half if small or in quarter

3. Cut your red onion, spring onion and garlic into dices and separate the layer.

4. In a large bowl, pour the chopped ingredient and add ½ cup of grain, 2tsp of black pepper, 2tsp thyme and parsley and gently mix thoroughly together.

5. For serving, transfer the salad onto a serving bowl. Dress with a desirable salad cream

6. Cover and refrigerate at least 1 hour before serving.

SALAD WITH VEGAN FETA CHEESE

Feta is the most well-known cheese in Greece. It is a soft, white, brined cheese that is very nutritious and an excellent calcium source. As part of Mediterranean cuisine, this cheese is used in all sorts of dishes ranging from appetizers to desserts. Vegan feta cheese has full nutrition facts.

Ingredients

1 medium English cucumber

8 cherry tomatoes

½ medium onion, peeled

8-10 iceberg lettuce, hand torn

½ cup whole green gram (sabut moongs) sprouts, steamed

Feta cheese as required

Dressing

3 tsps. mustard paste

2 tsps. lemon juice

1 tbsp dates paste

Rock salt (senda namak) to taste

Crushed black peppercorns to taste

Instructions

1. For the dressing, add the mustard paste in a bowl. Add lemon juice, dates paste, rock salt, crushed black peppercorns and mix well.

2. Cut the cucumber in triangles and cut the cherry tomatoes in halves. Cut the onion into dices and separate the layer.

3. Take lettuce in a large bowl, add the cut vegetables in it. Add green gram and 2 tbsps. Of the prepared dressing and gently toss.

4. For serving, transfer the salad on to a serving bowl. Crumble feta cheese and sprinkle on top.

PASTA SALAD

It serves as a good source of fiber, protein, healthy fats, and vitamin C. High in sodium. Pasta salad mainly contains carbs and fat, calories, net carbs, sugars, sodium, protein, total carbohydrates, and vitamins. If you are trying to choose healthy to side with your protein, choose a salad with a pasta side.

Ingredients

2 boxes of spelt penne

2 avocados cut in small pieces

1 1/2 cup of sun-dried tomatoes

1/2 cup of chopped onions

1/4 cup of almond milk

1/4 cup of fresh lime juice

3 tbs of maple syrup

4 tbs of sea salt

3-4 dashes of cilantro

1/2 cup of olive oil

Instructions

1. Cook the pasta as directed on the package

2. Add everything in a big bowl

3. Toss until evenly distributed

MUSHROOM SALAD

Mushrooms are a consumable organism that can give a few effective supplements. The numerous sorts of mushrooms have different arrangements and healthful profiles. Beyond the diet, mushrooms include in certain kinds of daily medication. Mushrooms contain protein, nutrients, minerals, and antioxidants. These can have different medical advantages. For instance, cell antioxidants are synthetic substances that help the body take out free extremists. Free extremists are poisonous results of digestion and other substantial cycles. They can aggregate in the body, and if too some gather, oxidative pressure can result. This can hurt the body's cells and may prompt different medical issues.

Among the cell antioxidant operators in mushrooms are Selenium, Vitamin C, Choline. Numerous sorts of mushrooms are consumable, and most give about similar amounts of similar supplements per serving, paying little mind to their shape or size.

Ingredients

1/4 bunch fresh spinach, torn	1/2 cup olive oil
1/4 bunch red leaf lettuce, torn	1/4 cup fresh lime juice
1/4 bunch romaine lettuce, torn	1/2 tsp. dill
1/2 lb. fresh mushrooms	1/2 tsp. basil
1/2 red bell pepper, chopped	1/2 tsp. sea salt
1 sm. red onion, diced	

Instructions

Thoroughly wash mushrooms, dry, slice

Add onion, bell pepper, olive oil, lime juice, dill, sea salt, and basil

Marinade 1/2 hour in refrigerator

Thoroughly wash greens, dry and shred

Place greens with mushrooms and mix thoroughly

VEGETABLE SALAD

Fresh vegetables give a cornucopia of goodness and assortment adds enthusiasm to your dinners. Make sure to turn these champs onto your staple eating routine rundown! Leafy vegetables usually are low in calories and fat and high in protein per calorie, dietary fiber, nutrient C, favorable to nutrient A carotenoid, folate, manganese and nutrient K. These plants are regularly considerably more productive than customary leaf vegetables, yet abuse of their rich nourishment is troublesome, because of their high fiber content. This can be overwhelmed by additional handling, for example, drying and granulating into powder or pulping and squeezing for juice.

Ingredients

1/2 lb. fresh string beans

(Remove ends and snap in half)

1/2 bunch romaine lettuce, torn

1/2 bunch watercress, torn

1/2 bunch cilantro, chopped fine

1/2 tsp. dill

1/4 tsp. cumin

Instructions

Put olive oil in a bowl

Add dill, cumin, basil, and lime juice

Marinade in refrigerator for 1-1/2 hours

Mix thoroughly with lettuce, watercress, and cilantro

DRESSING OF SALAD

AVOCADO DRESSING

Ingredients

3 Ripe avocados, peeled and seeded	1 tsp. chili powder
1/2 small red onion	1 tsp. oregano
1/2 tomato peeled	1 tsp. cumin
1/4 cup fresh lime juice	1/2 tsp. sweet basil
4 tbs pure olive oil	1/2 tsp. sweet basil
Pinch Cayenne Pepper	1/2 tsp. thyme
Few sprigs of cilantro	1/4 tsp. sea salt

Instructions

Pour avocados in blender

Add remaining ingredients and 2 tablespoons of spring water

Lightly blend and pour over your salad

Note: Season to taste

Use cold-pressed, virgin olive oil.

CREAMY SALAD DRESSING

Ingredients

4 tbs. almond butter	1/2 tsp. sweet basil
2 green onions	1/4 tsp. thyme
1/4 tsp. ground cumin	1 tsp. maple syrup
1/2 cup fresh lime juice	1/4 tsp. sea salt

Instructions

In a glass bottle, add all ingredients and 2 tablespoons of spring water

Shake thoroughly and enjoy!

CUCUMBER DRESSING

Ingredients

3 med. cucumbers, peeled	1/2 tsp. thyme
10 almonds, raw, unsalted	1/2 tsp. sea salt
4 tbs. pure olive oil	1/4 tsp. dill
1/4 cup fresh lime juice	1-1/2 cup spring water
1/4 cup green onions, chopped fine	Few sprigs of cilantro, choppe

Instructions

Blend 10 almonds in spring water, 2 minutes, high speed

Strain and set liquid aside

Puree cucumbers in blender with almonds

Add olive oil, lime juice and remaining ingredients

Lightly blend, adding liquid, if needed

Pour over your salad and enjoy!

XAVE'S DELIGHT

Ingredients

2 fresh limes squeezed

3 tbs. maple syrup

3 oz. sesame tahini

1 oz spring water

1 tsp. sea salt

1/2 tsp. red pepper

Instructions

In a glass bottle, add the juice of 2 limes, water, maple syrup, sea salt, red pepper, and sesame tahini.

Shake well and dress your salad!!

LIME AND OLIVE OIL DRESSING

Ingredients

1/4 fresh lime, squeezed

1/2 cup olive oil

1/8 cup spring water

1 tbs. maple syrup

1/4 tsp. sweet basil

1/4 tsp. thyme

1/4 tsp. oregano

1/4 tsp. ground cumin

Instructions

Put all ingredients in a glass bottle.

Shake thoroughly and enjoy this delicious and easy salad dressing!

SNACKS

MINT CHIP ENERGY BITES

Ingredients

1/8 teaspoon peppermint extricate

Touch of fine ocean salt

2 tablespoons smaller than usual chocolate chips

10 Medjool dates, pitted

½ cup of coconut chips

½ cup of hacked pecans

¼ cup of cocoa powder

Instructions

Add dates to your food processor and cycle until separated into pea-sized pieces.

Include coconut chips, pecans, cocoa powder, peppermint remove, also, a spot of salt and keep preparing until it is all around joined into a giant ball.

Fold the blend into about 1-inch balls and freeze for 20 minutes to move to the fridge.

NO-BAKE BROWNIE ENERGY BITES

Fixings Dry Ingredients:

½ cup without gluten oat flour

½ cup unsweetened cocoa powder

¼ cup ground flaxseed

½ cup veggie lover chocolate chips

Wet Ingredients:

¾ cup common, unsalted smooth almond spread

¼ cup unadulterated maple syrup

1 teaspoon unadulterated vanilla concentrate

Instructions

In a huge bowl, combine the entirety of the dry fixings: oat flour, cocoa powder, flaxseed and chocolate chips.

Add vanilla, maple syrup and almond spread while mixing and collapsing utilizing a spatula.

Utilizing a treat scoop, scoop and drop a ball into your hands.

Fold and press into chomps.

DAIRY-FREE BANANA NUT MUFFINS

Dry Ingredients:

1½ cups of without gluten oat flour

¾ cup of almond supper

¾ teaspoon of preparing powder

½ teaspoon of preparing pop

¼ teaspoon of salt

Wet Ingredients:

3 mediums, ready bananas (1 cup squashed)

¼ cup of liquefied coconut oil

¼ cup of coconut sugar

1 flax egg (1 tablespoon ground flax + 3 tablespoons water, whisk together, set for 15 mins)

1 teaspoon of unadulterated vanilla concentrat

Add-ins:

¾ cup pecans, cleaved

Discretionary for garnish

2 tablespoons pecans, cleaved

Instructions

Preheat the broiler to 350°F and fix a 12-cup biscuit skillet with biscuit liners.

Add striped bananas to a bowl and crush until they are smooth.

Rush in the flax egg, coconut oil, coconut sugar, and vanilla.

Keep rushing in oat flour, almond dinner, heating powder, preparing pop and salt until all-around consolidated at that point overlap in pecans.

Utilizing a huge scoop, scoop and drop hitter equitably into biscuit cups.

Prepare for around 20 minutes and put aside to cool on a cooling rack.

NO-BAKE SWEET POTATO CHOCOLATE CHIP COOKIES

Ingredients

A cup of dates hollowed and mollified

½ cup of smooth almond or cashew spread

½ cup of cooked and crushed or pureed yam

1 teaspoon of unadulterated vanilla concentrate

¼ teaspoon of cinnamon

A squeeze salt 7 to 8 tablespoons of natural coconut flour

1/3 cup of scaled down chocolate chips

Instructions

Add your dates to the bowl of a food processor and cycle on high until a glue structure.

When you accomplish the pale consistency, add the pounded sweet potato, nut margarine, vanilla, cinnamon and cycle until mixed.

Mix in 7 tablespoons of the coconut flour until a thick mixture structure, at that point, cool the mixture in the cooler for 20 minutes.

On the off chance that the mixture is still clingy, mix in some a greater amount of the coconut flour.

Crease in the smaller than usual chocolate chips and fold the batter into balls or then again treat shapes. They will have a treat batter like surface and are best put away in the fridge.

POTATO PANCAKES

Ingredients

2 chestnut potatoes, ground

1 enormous zucchini, ground

½ yellow onion, ground

½ cup of oat flour

A teaspoon of heating powder

½ teaspoon of newly ground dark pepper

Instructions

Preheat broiler to 420 degrees. Spread two sheet dishes with material paper.

Spread portion of the ground vegetables on a spotless kitchen towel, at that point roll and wring the towel to draw out the abundance dampness.

Move to an enormous blending bowl. Rehash with the excess vegetables.

In a little bowl, consolidate the oat flour, prepare powder, and pepper, add to the vegetable bowl, and blend well, utilizing your hands to circulate the flour and prepare powder equally.

Scoop a portion of the potato blend, and hand-shape it into a semi-tight ball. Level with your palms, and spot the flapjack onto the arranged dish. Rehash with the leftover blend, dividing the hotcakes properly.

Prepare for close to 15 minutes. Flip and heat for another 10 or more minutes. Top with your preferred topping.

MAIN COURSE RECIPES

POUNDED CAULIFLOWER AND GREEN BEAN CASSEROLE

Ingredients

¾ cup of coconut milk

½ cup of nourishing yeast

1 cauliflower

Salt and pepper to taste

14 ounces of green beans, managed

1 onion, diced

Instructions

In a skillet, cook cauliflower florets in vegetable stock and a few olive oil.

Include onions and beans and cook for somewhat more. Move the combination into a blender and add coconut milk, dietary yeast, salt also, pepper and mix until smooth.

In a preparing sheet, collect green bean blend, pounded cauliflower, also, garnishes and heat for 15 to 20 minutes at 400 degrees F.

BURRITO BOWL

Ingredients

Prepared tortilla chips

2 to 4 cups cooked grains

2 to 4 cups cooked beans

2 to 4 cups cleaved romaine lettuce or steamed kale

2 to 4 cleaved tomatoes

1 to 2 cleaved green onions

1 to 2 cups corn portions

1 avocado, cleaved

New salsa

Instructions

Break some tortilla chips and spot in a bowl.

Add some cooked grains and beans.

Layer on tomatoes, lettuce, corn, onions, avocado and afterward top with salsa.

ZUCCHINI NOODLES WITH PORTOBELLO BOLOGNESE

Ingredients

3 tablespoons additional virgin olive oil, separated

6 Portobello mushroom covers, stems, and gills eliminated and finely hacked

½ cup of minced carrot

½ cup of minced celery

½ cup of minced yellow onion

3 huge garlic cloves, minced

Legitimate salt

New ground pepper

1 tablespoon of tomato glue

A 28-ounce can squash tomatoes (I firmly suggest San Marzano)

2 teaspoons of dried oregano

¼ teaspoon of squashed red pepper (discretionary)

½ cup new basil leaves, finely hacked (in addition to extra for serving)

4 medium zucchinis

Instructions

Sauté garlic, mushrooms, celery, and carrots in olive oil in a skillet.

Season with salt and pepper as wanted. Keep cooking until vegetables are delicate.

Mix in some tomato glue and cook for a few minutes' prior adding squashed tomatoes, oregano, red pepper, and basil.

Let it stew for 10 to 15 minutes until the sauce thickens.

As the sauce stews, utilize a fitting sharp edge to make winding zucchini.

Sauté the zucchini noodles in a different pan for two or three minutes and season as wanted.

Top with a liberal measure of Bolognese and embellishment with newly cleaved basil and serve right away.

THAI NOODLES

Ingredients

8 ounces earthy colored rice noodles or other entire grain noodles

3 tablespoons of low-sodium soy sauce, or to taste

2 tablespoons of earthy colored rice syrup or maple syrup

2 tablespoons of new lime juice (from 1 to 2 limes)

4 garlic cloves, minced

3 cups of solidified Asian-style vegetables

1 cup of mung bean sprouts

2 green onions, white and light green parts hacked

3 tablespoons of hacked, cooked, unsalted peanuts

¼ cup of hacked new cilantro

1 lime, cut into wedges

Instructions

Adhere to directions for cooking noodles.

Consolidate soy sauce, garlic, earthy colored rice syrup, lime squeeze and cup water and heat to the point of boiling. Mix in the veggies and cook for around 5 minutes or until fresh delicate.

Add the cooked noodles and mung bean fledglings and throw to cover at that point let it cook for a couple more minutes.

Embellishment with cilantro, green onions, lime wedges and hacked peanuts.

MEDITERRANEAN VEGETABLE SPAGHETTI

Ingredients

10 ounces earthy colored rice spaghetti

1 red chime pepper, cubed little

1 yellow ringer pepper, cubed little

2 plum tomatoes, cut into eighths (dispose of the seeds)

Salt

½ jalapeño (discretionary)

2 tablespoons of dried spices de Provence

2 tablespoons of tomato purée

2 tablespoons apple juice vinegar or juice of 1 lime

12 cherry tomatoes, quartered

1 zucchini, divided at that point cut into meager half-adjusts

1 pack spinach, slashed

Small bunch of dark olives

Instructions

Cook pasta, channel and put in a safe spot.

Sauté peppers, tomatoes, jalapeno, and spices in a pot. Add water and let it stew.

Add tomato puree and vinegar or lime squeeze and let it cook together for a couple of moments until it gets sassy.

Add cherry tomatoes, zucchini cuts, and spinach. Blend well and cook for around 5 to 7 minutes.

Add olives and sauce to the pasts alongside certain spices.

MEXICAN LENTIL SOUP

Ingredients

2 tablespoons additional virgin olive oil

1 yellow onion, diced

2 carrots, stripped and diced

2 celery stems, diced

1 red ringer pepper, diced

3 cloves garlic, minced

1 tablespoon cumin

¼ teaspoon smoked paprika

1 teaspoon oregano

2 cups diced tomatoes and the juices

4 ounces diced green chilies

2 cups green lentils, flushed and picked over

8 cups vegetable stock

½ teaspoon salt

A scramble (or a greater amount of) hot sauce, in addition to additional for serving

New cilantro, for embellish

1 avocado, stripped, pitted, and diced, or embellish

Instructions

Sauté onions, celery, chime pepper and carrots in a prospect 5 minutes at that point add garlic, cumin, paprika, and oregano and let it cook for one more moment.

Include tomatoes, chilies, lentils, stock, and salt to taste and bring to a stew until lentils are delicate.

Season with salt and pepper as fundamental.

Serve it embellished with new cilantro, avocado, and a couple of runs of hot sauce.

PECAN MEAT TACOS

Ingredients Walnut Tacos:

1½ cups de-shelled pecans

1 teaspoon of garlic powder

½ teaspoon of cumin

½ teaspoon of stew powder

A tablespoon of tamari

6 Taco shells (natural and without gluten)

Fixings:

1 cup carrots hacked

1 cup red cabbage hacked

¼ cup of onion, hacked

Cilantro hacked

Lime Cashew Sour Cream:

1 Cup cashews splashed for the time being (or drenched in any event 10 mins in bubbling water)

½ cup of water (and more if necessary)

2 tablespoons of lime juice

A tablespoon of apple juice vinegar

Touch of salt to taste

Instructions

Mix pecans in a food processor until it looks "substantial."

Add pecans to a food processor and cycle until blend is thoughtful of "substantial."

Put blend in a bowl and add flavors and blend. Add the remaining fixings and mix well.

Fill taco shells with the combination and top as wanted.

Join all elements of the lime cashew sharp cream in a blender until smooth.

Top tacos with sharp cream.

PINEAPPLE PAPAYA FRIED RICE

Ingredients

3 cups of natural earthy colored rice, cooked and chilled

1 enormous papaya, stripped and cubed

A jar of 100% pineapple pieces just, channel the juice

½ cup of nursery peas (natural and neighborhood if conceivable)

1 cup of blended ringer peppers (green and sweet red)

1 medium measured onion, diced

3 little scallions, slashed

2 tsp of Coconut Aminos

3 garlic cloves, minced,

1 tsp of turmeric

1 tsp of new ginger, minced

½ teaspoon of Himalayan pink salt

1½ teaspoon of sesame seed oil

½ teaspoon of white pepper

2 tablespoons of coconut oil

1 teaspoon of thyme

Instructions

Soften coconut oil in a huge griddle and add turmeric, onion, scallion, garlic, and ginger.

Sauté until the onions are delicate at that point add ringer peppers and nursery peas.

Mix every so often until the veggies are delicate in surface.

Whenever this is accomplished, add papaya, pineapple and cold rice in the griddle and mix until the combination alternates yellow.

Sprinkle the coconut aminos and sesame oil into the griddle and flip on more than one occasion.

Season with thyme, white pepper, and salt and mix completely to develop the flavor. Serve as needs be.

GARLIC HASH BROWN WITH KALE

Ingredients

2 Yukon Gold potatoes, destroyed

¼ teaspoon salt

½ teaspoon of newly ground dark pepper

6 cloves garlic, minced

2 to 3 enormous kale leaves, destroyed

NOTE: You can substitute Yukon Gold potatoes with destroyed yams

Instructions

Preheat your stove to 375° F.

Season destroyed potatoes with salt and pepper and spread them on a preparing sheet fixed with a silicone heating mat and heat for 10 minutes.

Eliminate it from the stove and throw with minced garlic. Return them to the stove and heat for a couple more minutes.

In a huge container, over medium warmth, sauté destroyed kale with a few water until it is delicate and put aside to cool. Make a point not to add more water when it dissipates.

Press the kale to dispose of abundance water, and afterward throw it a piece to separate the cooked shreds.

Plate the crisped potatoes, top it with the kale, and serve.

CAULIFLOWER AND TOMATO COCONUT CURRY

Ingredients

1 yellow onion

4 cups of yam, cleaved

1 head cauliflower, cleaved

2 tablespoons of olive oil

1 teaspoon genuine salt, separated

2 tablespoons curry powder

1 tablespoon garam masala

1 teaspoon of cumin

¼ teaspoon of cayenne

23-ounce container of diced San Marzano plum tomatoes

A 15-ounce jar of coconut milk

A 15-ounce jar of chickpeas

4 cups of spinach leaves

Cilantro, for decorate

Earthy colored rice, for serving

Instructions

Cook earthy colored rice as trained.

Dice the onion and slash the yam into reduced down pieces (try not to strip). Slash the cauliflower into florets too.

Sauté onions in olive oil at that point add the yam and proceed cooking for 2 to 3 minutes.

Include cauliflower and salt to taste keep cooking for a couple more minutes. Presently, mix in curry powder, garam masala, cumin, cayenne, tomatoes and coconut milk.

Heat to the boiling point, and afterward let it stew for around 8 to 10 minutes until the cauliflower and yam are delicate.

Include chickpeas and spinach and mix a long time prior to preparing with salt as wanted.

Embellishment with hacked cilantro, and present with earthy colored rice.

DESSERT AND TREATS RECIPES

CREAM DECORATED TRUFFLES

Ingredients

For the truffles:

2 tablespoons of natural crude cacao

½ cup of natural crude zucchini

½ cup of moved oats

¼ cup Medjool dates or raisins

For the cream:

½ cup cashews

½ teaspoons of liquor free vanilla concentrate

2 Medjool dates, pitted

For brightening:

1 tablespoon separated water

½ tsp. natural crude cacao

Instructions

Consolidate truffle fixings in a blender until completely combined.

Utilizing wet hands structure the blend into little balls and put in a safe spot.

Consolidate cream fixings in a blender until smooth at that point spread it over a portion of the truffles.

Add two little pea size amounts of cream for the mummies' eyeballs for the excess truffles.

Blend water and cacao in a little bowl and utilize a toothpick to make drops of the combination onto the truffles.

CRUDE APPLE TART

Ingredients

3 natural apples (of your decision), ground

A cup of dried cranberries

A cup of antiquated moved oats

2 tablespoons of crude almond spread

1 cup of unsweetened coconut pieces

Instructions

Consolidate apples, cranberries, oats, and almond margarine in a dish.

Top with the coconut pieces, spread, and refrigerate for 2 hours.

CRUDE ORANGE CHOCOLATE PUDDING

Ingredients

1 vanilla bean, seeds scratched out (or 1 ½ tsp unadulterated vanilla concentrate)

A cup of stripped, pitted, and generally cleaved ready avocado

1 cup pitted dates

1/3 cup crude or customary cocoa powder

1 teaspoon of orange zing

½ cup of newly crushed squeezed orange

1/8 teaspoon of ocean salt

Instructions

Join all fixings in a food processor and puree until smooth.

You can thin the puree by adding more squeezed orange, or a sprinkle of nut milk or water.

Serve or store in the cooler.

MANGO CHIA SEED PUDDING

Ingredients

2 cups of coconut milk

½ cup of chia seeds

1 teaspoon of vanilla (powder or concentrate)

¼ teaspoon of cardamom

1 medium measured mango

3 tablespoons of coconut nectar or 2 tablespoons of date glue

Instructions

Blend chia seeds with coconut milk, coconut nectar, vanilla, and cardamom in a bowl and refrigerate up to expedite.

Cut the mango up into pieces and puree in a blender.

Serve in like manner – combine or serve in layers!

CHEWY LEMON AND OATMEAL COOKIES

Ingredients

10 dates, pitted

A cup of unsweetened fruit purée

1½ teaspoons of apple juice vinegar

A cup of moved oats

Some oat flours

½ cup brisk cooking oats

¾ cup generally slashed pecans

2 tablespoons of ground lemon zing (from around 2 lemons)

2 teaspoons of regular cocoa powder

1 teaspoon of vanilla powder

½ teaspoon of heating pop

Spot of ocean salt to taste

Instructions

Preheat the broiler to 275°F and fix 2 heating sheets with material paper.

Absorb the dates boiling water for around 20 minutes at that point mix them with fruit purée and vinegar.

Mix together the moved oats, oat flour, speedy cooking oats, pecans, lemon zing, cocoa powder, vanilla powder, preparing pop, also, salt in a huge bowl.

Blend in the dates and fruit purée glue and ensure that the blend is generally dry.

Scoop a part, fold it into a ball, pat it level and spot onto a preparing sheet. Rehash this until you go through the entire blend.

Prepare for around 40 minutes until the highest points of the treats show up firm and caramelized.

Let them cool on a wire rack.

CHOCOLATE BUCKWHEAT GRANOLA BARS

Ingredients

2 bananas

¼ cup of nutty spread (or almond margarine)

1 tablespoon of cocoa powder

1 teaspoon of all-common vanilla concentrate (I utilized my natively constructed one)

3 tablespoons of date syrup or maple syrup

1⅓ cup of buckwheat groats

⅓ - ½ cup of dull chocolate lumps (improved with solid sugars in the event that you can discover it or you can utilize unsweetened and increment the date syrup by 1 tablespoon)

Instructions

Preheat the stove to 360 degrees F (180 degrees Celsius).

Consolidate and pound the bananas with nutty spread, cocoa powder, vanilla concentrate and date syrup in a bowl.

Add chocolate and buckwheat groats and fill a brownie dish.

Prepare for around 20 minutes until the granola bars firm up then set it aside to cool.

CAULIFLOWER CHOCOLATE PUDDING

Ingredients

3 cups of cauliflower florets

2 cups of non-dairy milk (for example almond milk)

or a teaspoon of vanilla separate)

1/3 cup of cacao powder

10 pitted Medjool dates

½ teaspoon of vanilla bean powder (

Instructions

Steam the cauliflower until they become delicate.

Join all fixings in a blender until smooth and rich.

You can devour quickly or store in the cooler.

FIERY VEGAN BLACK BEAN BROWNIES

Ingredients

2 tablespoons of ground flax seed in addition to 6 tablespoons of water, blended well

1 cup (132 g) oat flour

1¼ cup (141 g) cacao or unsweetened cocoa powder

1 teaspoon of heating powder

1 teaspoon of finely ground ocean salt

2 teaspoons (5 g) of ground cinnamon

½ teaspoon cayenne powder (discretionary)

30 ounces (878 g) of cooked dark beans, depleted and flushed well

1 cup (240 ml) of unadulterated maple syrup

2 teaspoons (10 ml) of unadulterated vanilla concentrate

¼ (60 ml) cup water, add more by the teaspoon if necessary.

Instructions

Preheat the broiler to 350°F (176°C) and oil a container to make the flax eggs and let sit.

Add the oats, cocoa powder, heating powder, salt, cinnamon, and cayenne pepper to the food processor and granulate the oats into flour.

Whenever this has been done, include the beans, flax eggs, maple syrup, vanilla, and water and cycle until the hitter is smooth also, smooth. Use water to thin the blend as wanted.

Heat for thirty minutes and let it cool on a rack.

CHOCOLATE PEANUT BUTTER HIGH PROTEIN SUNDAE

Ingredients

1 banana, cut and solidified

½ cup of solidified cooked lentils

¼ cup of almond milk, or non-dairy milk of your decision

A tablespoon nutty spread

A tablespoon unsweetened cocoa powder

2 tablespoons of shelled, salted peanuts

2 teaspoons of cacao nibs

Instructions

Blend solidified banana cuts and lentils with almond milk, nut spread, and cocoa powder in a blender occasionally scratching the sides.

Serve in a bowl and top with peanuts and cacao nibs.

BERRY BASIL POPSICLES

Ingredients

1½ cup of cut strawberries

1 cup of blended berries (I utilized raspberry, red currant, and blueberry)

10 to 20 new basil leaves

A tablespoon of lemon juice

1 to 3 tablespoons of maple syrup (discretionary)

Instructions

Consolidate all fixings in a blender until smooth.

Empty the combination into Popsicle forms and supplement Popsicle sticks.

Freeze for the time being.

SMOOTHIES

INTRODUCTION

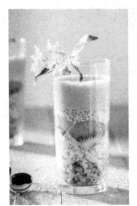

Smoothies are brimming with supplements and flavor. A nutritious breakfast gives a decent beginning to your day. It gives you energy to prop up throughout the day. In the summer, individuals worldwide search for mixed flavor approaches and great sustenance and get help from the burning warmth. Having smoothies with breakfast each day can certainly make ready for good wellbeing and pleasure all through the hot season. Smoothies are making with the new natural product. The heavenly taste and a ton of medical advantages make it a magnificent summer treat for your psyche and body. Smoothies cheer up your faculties as well as gang a colossal measure of health benefit.

21 IMPORTANT BENEFITS OF DRINKING HEALTHY SMOOTHIES HELPS YOU LOSE WEIGHT

Smoothies can help you lose excess body weight without skipping any meals. The fruits and berries used to prepare these drinks serve as excellent companions for keeping you healthy and feeling cooler on a hot summer morning. The enzymes present in several fruits help dissolve body fat and clear up your circulatory system.

PREVENTS DEHYDRATION

Water is the most plentiful thing both on earth and in your body. Around 70% of your body is water. Having smoothies alongside breakfast is an excellent method to recharge water loss in your body throughout the summer period.

MAKES YOU FEEL FULL

Individuals trying to lose weight frequently skirt the morning feast and wind up eating on food in bigger sums between suppers. To dodge this, specialists instruct having smoothies made regarding great leafy foods so you remain full for quite a while.

CONTROLS CRAVINGS

Smoothies are loaded with supplements and flavor. They are a fundamental piece essential in a best breakfast. As they give a force pressed beginning to the day. A ton of protein alongside numerous supplements curbs food longings and get you far from eating shoddy nourishment.

HELP IN EASY DIGESTION

Green smoothies that contain a ton of green verdant vegetables add basic nutrients and minerals to breakfast and help in assimilation. The fiber provided by these beverages duplicates the advantages of having a delectable breakfast, particularly throughout the mid-year.

WELLSPRING OF ANTIOXIDANTS

Green tea is a well-known wellspring of cancer prevention agents. You can add matcha green tea powder to make your smoothies wealthy in cell reinforcements, and these will help forestall a ton of illnesses. Grapes, berries and yams are regular wellsprings of cell reinforcements.

UPGRADES IMMUNITY

Invulnerability alludes to the capacity of your body to battle against microorganisms and sicknesses. This regular potential gets declined because of a few reasons. Curiously, having smoothies made of fixings that incorporate supplements like beta-carotene helps support your invulnerable framework.

CONTROLS SLEEP DISORDERS

Individuals having various age bunches far and wide regularly face issues identified with the absence of rest and fretfulness. A good breakfast joined by a smoothie made of bananas, kiwi and oats gives calcium and magnesium in great amounts. This incites rest and keeps up sound dozing designs.

IMPROVES SKIN

As you may know, food containing carotenoids, similar to mango and pumpkin, are profoundly gainful for skin and appearance. Hence, smoothies that contain these fixings assist you with continuing gleaming in the late spring.

GIVES LIQUID FOOD BENEFITS

Well-being and nourishment specialists overall recommend burning-through fluid nourishment for better absorption. Smoothies contain mixed soil products in fluid-structure that make it simpler for the body to separate them.

DETOXIFIES THE BODY

Nourishments like garlic, papaya and beets help purify your blood and dispose of a few poisons amassed in your body tissues. Hence to have an incredible breakfast you ought to incorporate smoothies as solid detoxifying drinks each day.

LIFTS BRAIN POWER

It is very apparent that that specific leafy foods increment mental aptitude and lift memory. Mental readiness and fixation are extraordinarily improved by fixings like coconut that are wealthy in omega-3 unsaturated fats. Smoothies with these fixings help the mind work quicker.

CONTROLS MOOD SWINGS

Natural leafy foods fill in as fantastic pressure busters. Smoothies made of new fixings ease pressure and assist you with remaining more joyful and more advantageous.

FIGHT DEPRESSION

New vegetables and organic products rich in folic corrosive, similar to broccoli, spinach and bananas, help keep despondency under control. Patients experiencing sadness are encouraged to eat well morning meals, and smoothies can be beneficial for them.

SUPPLIES CALCIUM

Normal admission of calcium in the perfect sum is fundamental for bone and tooth wellbeing. Also, it can influence hair development and heart working as well. Smoothies arranged with dairy or strengthened dairy options fill in as incredible wellsprings of calcium for the body.

CHECKS THE GROWTH OF CARCINOGENS

The development of disease-causing elements, or cancer-causing agents, can be checked by controlling free extremists' development in the body. Organic products like strawberries, blueberries and grapes are wealthy in cell reinforcements that restrain the development of malignant growth causing free revolutionaries.

GIVES A GOOD AMOUNT OF FIBER

The most widely recognized issue individuals experience the ill effects of today are identified with upset entrails. A decent measure of stringy food is basic for directing the excretory framework so you can appreciate summer without agonizing over your wellbeing. Smoothies with plenty of foods grown from the ground help keep your guts working easily.

IMPROVES BONE HEALTH

Calcium, nutrient D3 and nutrient K are supplements that improve bone wellbeing. Smoothies wealthy in these supplements contain spinach, green vegetables and citrus natural products as boss fixings. So, for the best breakfast in Edmond, you should attempt some cool smoothies that guarantee your bones remain sound for eternity.

FORESTALLS HEART DISORDERS

Coronary sicknesses, or illnesses identified with heart, require supplement rich food alongside proper prescription. Opportune breakfast that contains sans fat nourishments like oats and smoothies joined by customary practicing is the key for patients wishing to avoid heart issues.

HOLDS BLOOD SUGAR IN CHECK

High glucose and diabetes are the most widely recognized way of life illnesses that trouble individuals worldwide. Individuals who have imbalanced sugar levels in their blood are inclined to a few complexities. Having a morning meal that is wealthy in supplements but low in calories can make things simpler. Smoothies loaded with new soil products are able decisions to go for on blistering summer mornings, as they cause you to feel full and glad without expanding your sugar admission.

LESSENS CHANCES OF CANCER

A few wellbeing reports distributed overall propose that nourishments like cabbage, broccoli, and cauliflower are useful in battling against malignant growth. They assault free revolutionaries and accordingly forestall malignant growth. Smoothies made of these fixings demonstrate truly accommodating in forestalling disease development.

EQUILIBRIUMS HORMONAL FUNCTIONING

Hormones assume a huge part in managing our everyday capacities. Nonetheless, any lopsidedness in their different levels can prompt grave repercussions. Besides, a hormonal irregularity can welcome a few wellbeing risks. Consequently, to keep your hormones working easily, all you require is a reviving smoothie of your decision. This will cause you to feel cool and quiet this late spring.

Consider smoothies a consistently superior alternative over juice with regards to medical advantages. Juice is regularly liberated from the mash of leafy foods. Moreover, stripping natural products or vegetables prior to placing them into a juicer makes them inclined to germs and oxidation. Smoothies comprise all aspects of the fixings, securing all the integrity and healthiness of them.

PART FOUR

NUTRITIONAL GUIDE AND INTRODUCTION TO THE MEAL PLAN

THE ULTIMATE NUTRITIONAL GUIDE TO DR. SEBI'S DIET PLAN: THE GUIDELINE RULES TO FOLLOW ON DR. SEBI DIET

- You should never eat any foods which are not listed.

- Do not use a microwave, any canned foods, or any seedless fruits.

- No animal products, meat, fish, dairy, honey, white or brown sugars, and no alcohol.

- Drink as much spring water as possible.

- Eat cell food before taking medicines, sleep as much as possible, particularly during detoxing.

- Take Dr. Sebi's supplement one hour before western medicine.

A structured diet meal plan for a month can work wonders in record time when focusing on getting a balanced diet to your system continually. This particular process can ignite the efforts of the various weight loss functions and other necessary disease treatment going on in your body. All bodies naturally can do this. Switching to eating like this on a monthly basis can show you how quickly you can turn around the state of health in your body, your energy levels, and drop pounds from your frame. Adopting this kind of meal plan for a month may just appeal to you in a fashion that disables you from going back to a thoughtless, "eat what I want, eat when I want" mantra. The overall benefits can be shocking and effective.

MONTHLY PLAN

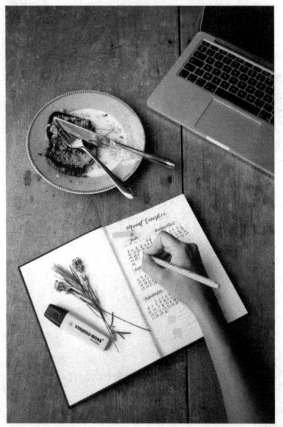

The right meal plans on a monthly basis should include a balanced array of vegetables that you like, and maybe some that you don't. When you simply eat what you always eat and do what you always do you will have the same body that you always have had. Not only that you will find out as you get older, but you will also need to do more for your body if you choose to maintain it in a healthy way. With age, our metabolism naturally slows down. People have shown that with these eating practices and with regular exercise that we can do a lot to offset these natural occurrences. Without the proper meal plan to reduce weight, then chances are you are not getting all the necessary fundamental nutrients that this type of method will naturally provide.

For effective weekly meal planning, you will need to take into consideration that protein will need to be delivered constantly throughout the day. Ready reserves of your favorite protein staples should always be ready.

When planning on eating more fruits and vegetables, make sure you are not mixing the old stuff with the new stuff. Try and make it a habit to clean out the fridge with the old stuff, and replace them with the new. Incorporating old foods with the new can ruin meal plans, and put a sour on a treat that you thought you were going to enjoy. It can also stifle your meal schedule, and force you to go into your other food reserves once again.

Fruits are naturally sweet with natural crabs, and most do not have a very high level of sugar to spike blood sugar levels out of proportion. Fruits also have water and fiber, two more natural things that your body will need for these things to happen properly.

Are you in search of a daily or monthly meal plan but can't seem to find highly effective ones that work for you? It's your lucky time!

Look this book:

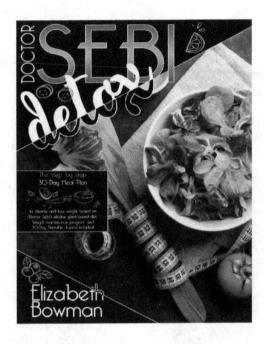

"Dr. Sebi Detox: The step by step 30-Day Meal Plan to cleanse and lose weight based on Doctor Sebi's alkaline plant-based diet. Weight maintenance program and 30-Day Printable Journal included!" by *Elizabeth Bowman*

In this book, you can find 30-day meal plan ideas concordant with Dr. Sebi's diet and recommendations. Meal planning is a great insight to enforce that you and your family maintain healthy eating habits.

You will never run out of dish ideas with this large collection of meal plans. The possibilities are endless! Let your creativity and cooking experience guide you. Your favorite 30-day-long meal plan is right around the corner.

CONCLUSIONS

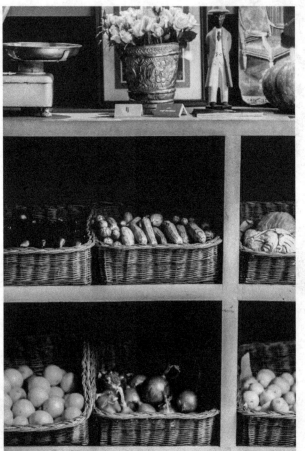

We as an individual realize that eating out can be challenging when trying to follow an entire food, plant-based diet and maintaining a strategic distance from oil and other concentrated fixings or on the off chance that you have to eat without gluten as recommended by Dr. Sebi. Then again, requesting takeout or dine-in can be quite convenient after a long, stressed, and hectic day where processed food was basically not in your arrangements. In this way, here are a few tips you can utilize when eating out.

Look into specialty restaurants, for example, plant-based eateries or vegetarian restaurants.

Determine how you need your dinners arranged. Always opt for steamed, heated, water sautéed or barbecued

Get along with the stand by staff to get them to cause your inclinations to occur.

It's clear now to see how a plant-based diet's way of life can be advantageous for your health rather than proceed with a vegan diet. I trust that the book addressed all inquiries you may have caught wind of this way of slimming down and that you can begin to make it work for you. If you are as yet reluctant about completely surrendering animal products, you don't need to. The fundamental remove here is that you make plant-based supreme principle part of your diet as you make gradual steps to progress into a full plant-based way of life. You will soon understand that your body and mind begin to feel good, stronger, healthier, and more advantageous. You can't fix your wellbeing until you fix your diet!

A good mindset is important, but you need to make sure that you are fully informed. This can be achieved by understanding what good food choices are; the best way to achieve this by researching the subject. For example, reading every book can get hold of on the library's low carbohydrate diet lifestyle. Surfing the net, by typing into the search engine the words, low carbohydrate diets, then visiting the blogs and websites that come up in the search.

Develop and cultivate new healthy eating habits. These can include eating regular meals and fewer snacks and preparing most meals at home rather than eating in restaurants or eating from fast food outlets. Try monitoring your intake by counting carbs.

Think of strategies you could use to tackle stress and other emotional problems in ways that do not involve food or drink. It may be that you have turned to food throughout your life to help you cope through difficult or stressful times. For example, you could try expressing your feelings by talking to somebody, instead of internalizing your emotions and turning to food.

Find ways of increasing the amount of exercise you get during the day. These could be as simple as walking up stairs instead of taking the elevator, taking the dogs out for walks, taking the kids to the park, walk instead of taking the car for short trips. You may also want to consider organized exercise. Perhaps joining a gym or taking up yoga, exercise classes, or dance classes.

Losing weight on a low carbohydrate diet can be relatively easy, but what happens when we finish the diet? You are now left trying to maintain the bodyweight you are comfortable with. It is so easy to go back to old habits, and ways of eating that will result in you putting the pounds back on. I believe it is those people that make an effort to develop strategies to organize and plan their daily diet who are going to be those who will have the most success at maintaining their weight.

The single most effective strategy to develop is your mindset, making or breaking your continuing maintenance diet after losing weight. Ultimately your success will depend on what is going on in your mind. Weight gain is often more about what goes on in your mind than what goes into your mouth.

Measure your performance. This can be done by weighing yourself regularly. I like to weigh myself every day, but you may prefer to weigh weekly. There are other ways of tracking your performance; for example, if you don't want to weigh yourself, you could instead see how comfortably you fit into a pair of trousers or skirt that is your maintenance target size. Another alternative to weighing yourself is to measure your waist using a tape measure frequently. The method you use to monitor your weight does not matter, and the important thing is to measure your performance regularly.

Use charts, trackers, and meal planners to record your performance and goals, which will help keep you motivated and on target. When I weigh myself daily, I quickly jot the weight down on a calendar I have hanging on the wall.

That's why I decided to give you a great and useful gift!

At the end of this book you'll find included:

"Dr. Sebi Journal: 30 Days to Detox and Improve Yourself. In this motivation journal based on Dr. Sebi's plant-based alkaline diet, you can keep track of your meals, goals, and progress" by *Elizabeth Bowman*, a 30-day based journal where you can write down all of your steps to wellness and detoxification.

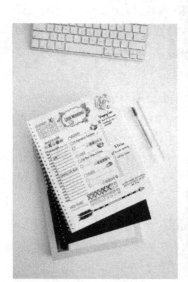
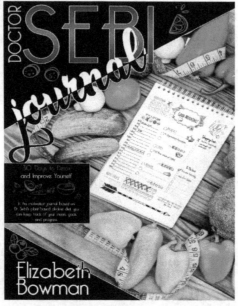
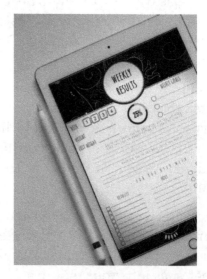

You'll be able to write down all of your daily meals, shopping list, thoughts, goals, and successes.

You will find inside all the instructions to do so.

You'll be able to fill out your daily plan directly in the book or download a printable version at the link you see below to use the planner all year round as well.

https://ebowmanwriter.wixsite.com/doctorsebi

I hope that by following some of my suggestions, you will be successful in maintaining your weight. Following a low carbohydrate maintenance diet and follow the food recommended by Dr. Sebi, can be an excellent way to maintain your body at the weight you want. I wish you every success.

ABOUT THE AUTHOR

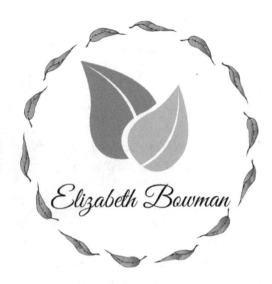

BIOGRAPHY

Elizabeth Bowman is an American author born and raised in the great state of Texas. While stumbling around in search of her true course in life she began to notice the state of those around her.

Everywhere she went Elizabeth noticed masses of people with obviously unhealthy lifestyles. She went back to college and earned a Bachelors in Dietetics from Baylor University.

Elizabeth spent several years working in different practices before opening her own business. Her one passion in life is from helping others achieve their weight-loss goals while retraining their minds to enjoy a cleaner, healthy existence.

Elizabeth specializes in alternative diets with an emphasis on vegan. She has tailored her programs to include the total package, with focuses on losing weight and keeping it off, and a combination of mental health and physical wellbeing.

Her bestselling book, Dr. Sebi Diet: Plant Based Meal Plan for Sustainable Weight Loss. Detox Your Body with Healthy Lifestyle Based Diets and Boost Your Energy Through the Day is available everywhere.

Her belief that having knowledge is only as important as sharing it is conveyed in all she does. Elizabeth is generous and caring, showing genuine concern for her patients as she helps them traverse the often difficult course back to better health.

She has helped thousands of patients over the course of her career and plans to continue until Father Time gets the better of her.

Elizabeth is the proud mother of two adult women and a devoted wife of over thirty years. To relax and unwind she enjoy long walks with her husband and their dogs, yoga, meditation, and reading. The inspiration for clean living prompted her to seek out innovative and unique recipes for the whole family.

BOOKS BY ELIZABETH BOWMAN

- 2020
  - o *Dr. Sebi Diet: Plant-Based Meal Plan for Sustainable Weight-Loss. Detox Your Body with Healthy Lifestyle Based Diets and Boost Your Energy Through the Day*
- 2021
  - o *Dr. Sebi Diet: The complete guide to the Sebi Plant-Based Diet. How to eliminate mucus from your body, detox and prevent disease with alkaline food list. 2021 Edition with 30-Day Printable Journal!*
  - o *Dr. Sebi Detox: The step by step 30-Day Meal Plan to cleanse and lose weight based on Doctor Sebi's alkaline plant-based diet. Weight maintenance program and 30-Day Printable Journal included!*
  - o *Dr.Sebi Journal: 30 Days to Detox and Improve Yourself. In this motivation journal based on Dr. Sebi's plant-based alkaline diet, you can keep track of your meals, goals, and progress.*

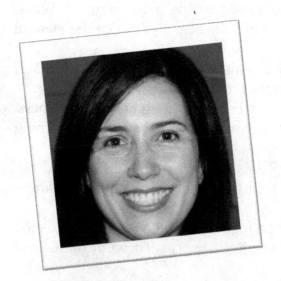

"…Hi I'm Elizabeth!

*I live through the publication of my books, if you liked this guide, I invite you to write an **honest review** and visit my author page on Amazon site.*

Thank you"

Elizabeth Bowman

PART FIVE

DR. SEBI JOURNAL

30 DAYS TO DETOX AND IMPROVE YOURSELF. IN THIS MOTIVATION JOURNAL BASED ON DR. SEBI'S PLANT-BASED ALKALINE DIET, YOU CAN KEEP TRACK OF YOUR MEALS, GOALS, AND PROGRESS.

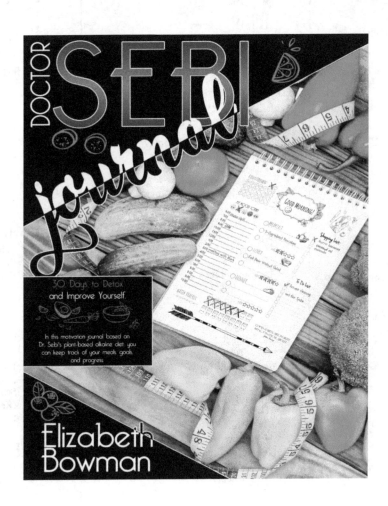

✂ **STICK IT ON THE FRIDGE!**

NUTRITIONAL GUIDE

- If a food is not listed in this Nutritional Guide, it is NOT recommended.
- Drink one gallon of natural spring water daily.
- Take Dr. Sebi's products one hour before pharmaceuticals.
- All of Dr. Sebi's products may be taken together with no interaction.
- Following the Nutritional Guide strictly and taking the products regularly produces the best results with reversing disease.
- No animal products, no dairy, no fish, no hybrid foods and no alcohol.

- Natural growing grains are alkaline-based; it is recommended that you consume only the grains listed in the Nutritional Guide instead of wheat.
- Many of the grains listed in the Nutritional Guide are available as pasta, bread, flour or cereal and can be purchased at better health food stores.
- Dr. Sebi's products are still releasing therapeutic properties 14 days after being taken.
- Dr. Sebi says, *"Avoid using a microwave, it will kill your food."*
- Dr. Sebi says, *"No canned or seedless fruits"*

Vegetables

- Amaranth greens (Callaloo, a variety of greens)
- Avocado
- Bell Peppers
- Chayote (Mexican squash)
- Cucumber
- Dandelion greens
- Garbanzo beans
- Izote (Cactus flower/cactus leaf)
- Kale
- Lettuce (All, except Iceberg)
- Mushrooms (All, except Shitake)
- Nopales (Mexican cactus)
- Okra
- Olives
- Onions
- Sea Vegetables (Wakame/dulse/arame/hijiki/nori)
- Squash
- Tomato (Cherry and plum only)
- Tomatillo
- Turnip greens
- Zucchini
- Watercress
- Purslane (Verdolaga)
- Wild arugula

Natural Herbal Teas

- Burdock
- Chamomile
- Elderberry
- Fennel
- Ginger
- Raspberry
- Tila

Fruits

- Apples (Granny Smith and Red delicious not recommended)
- Bananas (The smallest one or the Burro/midsize/original banana)
- Berries (All varieties, no cranberries)
- Elderberries (In any form)
- Cantaloupe
- Cherries
- Currants
- Dates
- Figs
- Grapes (Seeded)
- Limes (Key limes, with seeds)

Grains

- Amaranth
- Fonio
- Kamut
- Quinoa
- Rye
- Spelt
- Tef
- Wild Rice

Nuts & Seeds

- Hemp Seeds
- Raw Sesame Seeds
- Raw Sesame "Tahini" Butter
- Walnuts
- Brazil Nuts

Oils

- Olive Oil (Do not cook)
- Coconut Oil (Do not cook)
- Grapeseed Oil
- Sesame Oil
- Hempseed Oil
- Avocado Oil

Mild Flavors

- Basil
- Bay Leaf
- Cloves
- Dill
- Oregano
- Savory
- Sweet Basil
- Tarragon
- Thyme

Pungent and Spicy Flavors

- Achiote
- Cayenne/ African Bird Pepper
- Coriander (Cilantro)
- Onion Powder
- Habanero
- Sage

Salty Flavors

- Pure Sea Salt
- Powdered Granulated Seaweed
- (Kelp/Dulse/Nori – has "sea taste")

Sweet Flavors

- Pure Agave Syrup (From cactus)
- Date Sugar

HOW TO COMPILE THE "DETOX DAILY DIARY"

COMPILING THE JOURNAL IN ALL PARTS IS VERY IMPORTANT FOR YOUR PHYSICAL AND MENTAL DEVELOPMENT.
KEEPING TRACK OF YOUR THOUGHTS, PROGRESS, AND EVEN YOUR DELUSIONS WILL HELP YOU UNDERSTAND YOUR SELF'S CHANGES.

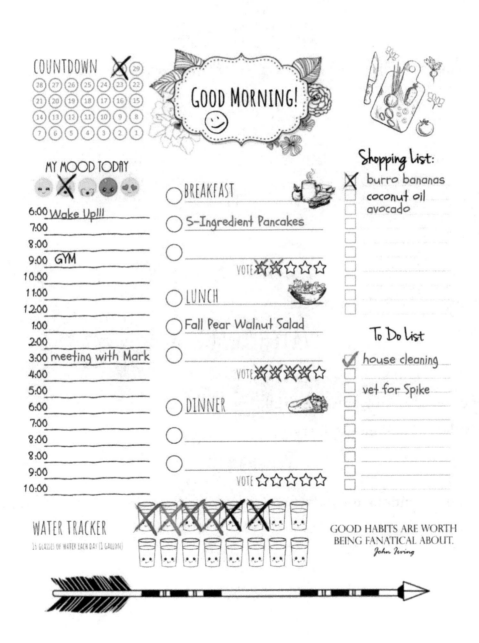

DAILY DIARY INSTRUCTIONS

COUNTDOWN

As you begin your journey the 30-day countdown to complete detoxification will begin.

You can use this "undated daily planner" at any point of the year.

SHOPPING LIST

in this section, you can write down all the ingredients you will need to prepare the day's meals and compile a shopping list.

MEAL PLANNER

Use this space to plan or log your daily meals and snacks easily

VOTE

Rate your recipes

NOTES

write the negative and positive aspects of the day

WATER TRACKER

Drinking water is essential!

Keep track of every glass of water you drink.

16 glasses of water = 1 gallon =3.8 liters

TO DO LIST

Think about your intentions for today and tomorrow, note them down so you don't forget anything

CITATIONS

Here you will find some quotes that will help you in your journey

WEEKLY RESULTS INSTRUCTIONS

At the end of each week record all your progress on the physical and mental detox plan.

Check and track your weight.

Think about the past week, identify your goals, and analyze the behaviors that you can improve.

Target your priorities for the following week.

MONTHLY RESULTS INSTRUCTIONS

At the end of 30 days you will have completed your detoxification program.

Check and track your weight.

Review the past month and record your goals.

Compare your results with the information that you wrote on the "presentation page" 30 days ago.

Only in this way will you be able to understand the real benefits you have

achieved for your physical and mental health.

HOW TO PRINT THE PLANNER

You can either print directly by clicking on the printer icon or save the planner on your PC and print from the file..

When printing directly from the app, check the print preview before you print. If the printable does not fit on the page then change the settings until it does fit (for example, click on "fit on page" if your browser has that option).

Alternatively, just download the file and open it to print.

If you cannot print directly (for example if you have a popup blocker installed on your PC) then just download the file and print from your PC.

LET'S GO !!!

NAME _____

GENDER _____

AGE _____

HEIGHT _____

WEIGHT _____

0%

PHYSICAL DISEASES

☐ _____
☐ _____
☐ _____
☐ _____
☐ _____
☐ _____
☐ _____
☐ _____

WHAT ARE YOUR GOALS? WHAT WOULD YOU LIKE TO IMPROVE?

MIND   BODY

SUNDAY	MONDAY	TUESDAY	WEDNESDAY	THURSDAY	FRIDAY	SATURDAY	NOTES

0	1	2	3	4	5	6	7
8	9	10	11	12	13	14	15
16	17	18	19	20	21	22	23
24	25	26	27	28	29	30

Stay **determined**

COUNTDOWN

(30) (29)
(28) (27) (26) (25) (24) (23) (22)
(21) (20) (19) (18) (17) (16) (15)
(14) (13) (12) (11) (10) (9) (8)
(7) (6) (5) (4) (3) (2) (1)

GOOD MORNING!

MY MOOD TODAY

6:00 _____
7:00 _____
8:00 _____
9:00 _____
10:00 _____
11:00 _____
12:00 _____
1:00 _____
2:00 _____
3:00 _____
4:00 _____
5:00 _____
6:00 _____
7:00 _____
8:00 _____
8:00 _____
9:00 _____
10:00 _____

○ BREAKFAST
○ _____
○ _____
VOTE ☆☆☆☆☆

○ LUNCH
○ _____
○ _____
VOTE ☆☆☆☆☆

○ DINNER
○ _____
○ _____
VOTE ☆☆☆☆☆

Shopping List:

☐
☐
☐
☐
☐
☐
☐
☐
☐
☐
☐

To Do list

☐
☐
☐
☐
☐
☐
☐
☐
☐
☐
☐

WATER TRACKER

16 GLASSES OF WATER EACH DAY (1 GALLON)

GOOD HABITS ARE WORTH
BEING FANATICAL ABOUT.
John Irving

133

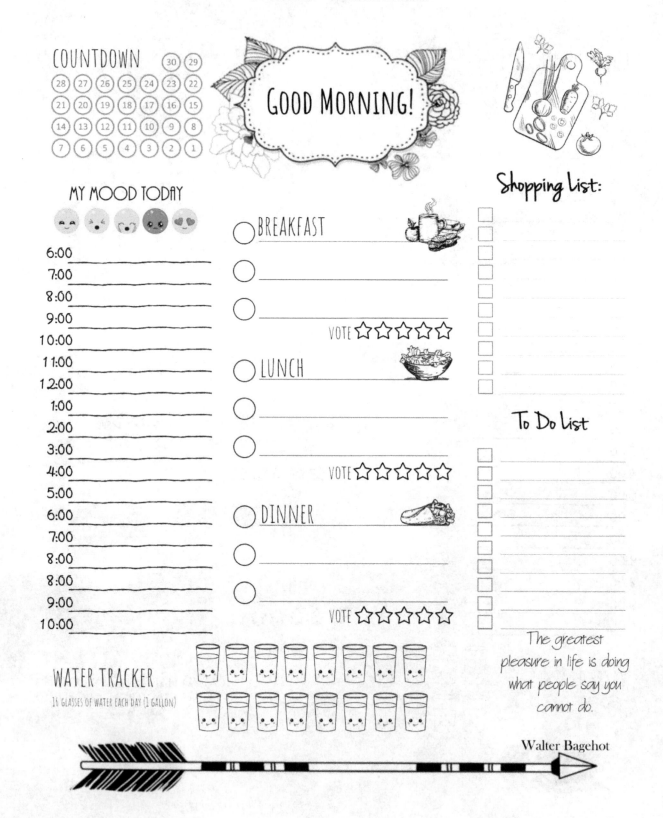

COUNTDOWN

30 29
28 27 26 25 24 23 22
21 20 19 18 17 16 15
14 13 12 11 10 9 8
7 6 5 4 3 2 1

GOOD MORNING!

Shopping List:

MY MOOD TODAY

6:00
7:00
8:00
9:00
10:00
11:00
12:00
1:00
2:00
3:00
4:00
5:00
6:00
7:00
8:00
8:00
9:00
10:00

BREAKFAST

VOTE ☆☆☆☆☆

LUNCH

VOTE ☆☆☆☆☆

DINNER

VOTE ☆☆☆☆☆

To Do list

The greatest pleasure in life is doing what people say you cannot do.

Walter Bagehot

WATER TRACKER

16 GLASSES OF WATER EACH DAY (1 GALLON)

134

COUNTDOWN

30 29 28 27 26 25 24 23 22 21 20 19 18 17 16 15 14 13 12 11 10 9 8 7 6 5 4 3 2 1

GOOD MORNING!

Shopping List:

MY MOOD TODAY

6:00
7:00
8:00
9:00
10:00
11:00
12:00
1:00
2:00
3:00
4:00
5:00
6:00
7:00
8:00
8:00
9:00
10:00

○ BREAKFAST
○
○
VOTE ☆☆☆☆☆

○ LUNCH
○
○
VOTE ☆☆☆☆☆

○ DINNER
○
○
VOTE ☆☆☆☆☆

To Do list

WATER TRACKER
16 GLASSES OF WATER EACH DAY (1 GALLON)

DON'T expect
to see a
CHANGE
YOU DON'T
if
make one

135

COUNTDOWN

30 29
28 27 26 25 24 23 22
21 20 19 18 17 16 15
14 13 12 11 10 9 8
7 6 5 4 3 2 1

GOOD MORNING!

MY MOOD TODAY

6:00 _____
7:00 _____
8:00 _____
9:00 _____
10:00 _____
11:00 _____
12:00 _____
1:00 _____
2:00 _____
3:00 _____
4:00 _____
5:00 _____
6:00 _____
7:00 _____
8:00 _____
8:00 _____
9:00 _____
10:00 _____

○ BREAKFAST
○ _____
○ _____
VOTE ☆☆☆☆☆

○ LUNCH
○ _____
○ _____
VOTE ☆☆☆☆☆

○ DINNER
○ _____
○ _____
VOTE ☆☆☆☆☆

Shopping List:
☐ _____
☐ _____
☐ _____
☐ _____
☐ _____
☐ _____
☐ _____
☐ _____
☐ _____

To Do list
☐ _____
☐ _____
☐ _____
☐ _____
☐ _____
☐ _____
☐ _____
☐ _____
☐ _____

THE FIRST STEP TO GETTING
ANYWHERE IS DECIDING
THAT YOU NO LONGER
WANT TO STAY WHERE
YOU ARE.

WATER TRACKER
16 GLASSES OF WATER EACH DAY (1 GALLON)

COUNTDOWN

30 29
28 27 26 25 24 23 22
21 20 19 18 17 16 15
14 13 12 11 10 9 8
7 6 5 4 3 2 1

GOOD MORNING!

Shopping List:

MY MOOD TODAY

6:00 _____
7:00 _____
8:00 _____
9:00 _____
10:00 _____
11:00 _____
12:00 _____
1:00 _____
2:00 _____
3:00 _____
4:00 _____
5:00 _____
6:00 _____
7:00 _____
8:00 _____
8:00 _____
9:00 _____
10:00 _____

○ BREAKFAST _____
○ _____
○ _____
VOTE ☆☆☆☆☆

○ LUNCH _____
○ _____
○ _____
VOTE ☆☆☆☆☆

○ DINNER _____
○ _____
○ _____
VOTE ☆☆☆☆☆

To Do List

WATER TRACKER
16 GLASSES OF WATER EACH DAY (1 GALLON)

Do what you **have to do** *until* you can do what you **want to do**

Oprah Winfrey

137

COUNTDOWN

30 29
28 27 26 25 24 23 22
21 20 19 18 17 16 15
14 13 12 11 10 9 8
7 6 5 4 3 2 1

GOOD MORNING!

MY MOOD TODAY

6:00 _____
7:00 _____
8:00 _____
9:00 _____
10:00 _____
11:00 _____
12:00 _____
1:00 _____
2:00 _____
3:00 _____
4:00 _____
5:00 _____
6:00 _____
7:00 _____
8:00 _____
8:00 _____
9:00 _____
10:00 _____

○ BREAKFAST

○ _____
○ _____

VOTE ☆☆☆☆☆

○ LUNCH

○ _____
○ _____

VOTE ☆☆☆☆☆

○ DINNER

○ _____
○ _____

VOTE ☆☆☆☆☆

Shopping List:

☐
☐
☐
☐
☐
☐
☐
☐
☐
☐

To Do list

☐
☐
☐
☐
☐
☐
☐
☐
☐
☐

WATER TRACKER

16 GLASSES OF WATER EACH DAY (1 GALLON)

YOU ONLY **fail**
WHEN *you*
STOP trying

COUNTDOWN

30 29
28 27 26 25 24 23 22
21 20 19 18 17 16 15
14 13 12 11 10 9 8
7 6 5 4 3 2 1

GOOD MORNING!

Shopping List:

☐
☐
☐
☐
☐
☐
☐
☐
☐
☐
☐

MY MOOD TODAY

6:00 _____
7:00 _____
8:00 _____
9:00 _____
10:00 _____
11:00 _____
12:00 _____
1:00 _____
2:00 _____
3:00 _____
4:00 _____
5:00 _____
6:00 _____
7:00 _____
8:00 _____
8:00 _____
9:00 _____
10:00 _____

○ BREAKFAST _____
○ _____
○ _____
VOTE ☆☆☆☆☆

○ LUNCH _____
○ _____
○ _____
VOTE ☆☆☆☆☆

○ DINNER _____
○ _____
○ _____
VOTE ☆☆☆☆☆

To Do list

☐
☐
☐
☐
☐
☐
☐
☐
☐
☐
☐

LIVE AS IF YOU WERE TO
DIE TOMORROW.
LEARN AS IS YOU WERE
TO LIVE FOREVER.

Mahatma Gandhi

WATER TRACKER
16 GLASSES OF WATER EACH DAY (1 GALLON)

WEEKLY RESULTS

WEEK [1] [2] [3] [4]

WEIGHT _____

LOST WEIGHT _____

25%

WEEKLY GOALS

○ _____
○ _____
○ _____

CHECK YOUR GOALS FOR THE PAST WEEK. ARE YOU SATISFIED?
GIVE YOURSELF AN HONEST RATING ON A SCALE OF 1 TO 10.

_____
_____
_____

WHAT DID YOU DO AND WHAT COULD YOU BETTER?

_____
_____
_____
_____

- FOR THE NEXT WEEK -

TO DO LIST

☐ _____
☐ _____
☐ _____
☐ _____
☐ _____
☐ _____
☐ _____
☐ _____
☐ _____

NOTES

_____
_____
_____
_____
_____
_____
_____

TOP 3 PRIORITIES

○ _____
○ _____
○ _____

**YOU ONLY fail
WHEN you
STOP trying**

COUNTDOWN

30 29
28 27 26 25 24 23 22
21 20 19 18 17 16 15
14 13 12 11 10 9 8
7 6 5 4 3 2 1

GOOD MORNING!

MY MOOD TODAY

6:00
7:00
8:00
9:00
10:00
11:00
12:00
1:00
2:00
3:00
4:00
5:00
6:00
7:00
8:00
8:00
9:00
10:00

○ BREAKFAST

○ _____

○ _____

VOTE ☆☆☆☆☆

○ LUNCH

○ _____

○ _____

VOTE ☆☆☆☆☆

○ DINNER

○ _____

○ _____

VOTE ☆☆☆☆☆

Shopping List:

To Do List

Life isn't about finding yourself. Life is about creating yourself.

George Bernard Shaw

WATER TRACKER

16 GLASSES OF WATER EACH DAY (1 GALLON)

COUNTDOWN

30 29
28 27 26 25 24 23 22
21 20 19 18 17 16 15
14 13 12 11 10 9 8
7 6 5 4 3 2 1

GOOD MORNING!

MY MOOD TODAY

6:00 _____
7:00 _____
8:00 _____
9:00 _____
10:00 _____
11:00 _____
12:00 _____
1:00 _____
2:00 _____
3:00 _____
4:00 _____
5:00 _____
6:00 _____
7:00 _____
8:00 _____
8:00 _____
9:00 _____
10:00 _____

○ BREAKFAST
○ _____
○ _____
VOTE ☆☆☆☆☆

○ LUNCH
○ _____
○ _____
VOTE ☆☆☆☆☆

○ DINNER
○ _____
○ _____
VOTE ☆☆☆☆☆

Shopping List:

☐
☐
☐
☐
☐
☐
☐
☐
☐
☐

To Do list

☐
☐
☐
☐
☐
☐
☐
☐
☐
☐

WATER TRACKER
16 GLASSES OF WATER EACH DAY (1 GALLON)

Be stronger than your excuses

142

COUNTDOWN

30 29
28 27 26 25 24 23 22
21 20 19 18 17 16 15
14 13 12 11 10 9 8
7 6 5 4 3 2 1

Good Morning!

MY MOOD TODAY

6:00
7:00
8:00
9:00
10:00
11:00
12:00
1:00
2:00
3:00
4:00
5:00
6:00
7:00
8:00
8:00
9:00
10:00

○ BREAKFAST

○
○

VOTE ☆☆☆☆☆

○ LUNCH

○
○

VOTE ☆☆☆☆☆

○ DINNER

○
○

VOTE ☆☆☆☆☆

Shopping List:

To Do list

WATER TRACKER

16 GLASSES OF WATER EACH DAY (1 GALLON)

LIFE BEGINS AT THE END OF YOUR COMFORT ZONE.

COUNTDOWN

30 29
28 27 26 25 24 23 22
21 20 19 18 17 16 15
14 13 12 11 10 9 8
7 6 5 4 3 2 1

GOOD MORNING!

Shopping List:

☐
☐
☐
☐
☐
☐
☐
☐
☐
☐

MY MOOD TODAY

○ BREAKFAST

_____

_____

VOTE ☆☆☆☆☆

6:00 _____
7:00 _____
8:00 _____
9:00 _____
10:00 _____
11:00 _____

○ LUNCH

12:00 _____
1:00 _____
2:00 _____
3:00 _____

_____

_____

VOTE ☆☆☆☆☆

4:00 _____
5:00 _____

To Do List

☐
☐
☐
☐

○ DINNER

6:00 _____
7:00 _____

_____

☐
☐
☐

8:00 _____

_____

☐
☐

8:00 _____
9:00 _____

VOTE ☆☆☆☆☆

☐
☐
☐

10:00 _____

WATER TRACKER

16 GLASSES OF WATER EACH DAY (1 GALLON)

Don't **STOP**
UNTIL
you're
PROUD

144

COUNTDOWN

30 29
28 27 26 25 24 23 22
21 20 19 18 17 16 15
14 13 12 11 10 9 8
7 6 5 4 3 2 1

GOOD MORNING!

MY MOOD TODAY

6:00
7:00
8:00
9:00
10:00
11:00
12:00
1:00
2:00
3:00
4:00
5:00
6:00
7:00
8:00
8:00
9:00
10:00

○ BREAKFAST
○
○
VOTE ☆☆☆☆☆

○ LUNCH
○
○
VOTE ☆☆☆☆☆

○ DINNER
○
○
VOTE ☆☆☆☆☆

Shopping List:

To Do list

WATER TRACKER
16 GLASSES OF WATER EACH DAY (1 GALLON)

Knowing is not enough. We must apply. Willing is not enough. We must do.

Bruce Lee

145

COUNTDOWN

30 29
28 27 26 25 24 23 22
21 20 19 18 17 16 15
14 13 12 11 10 9 8
7 6 5 4 3 2 1

Good Morning!

Shopping List:

MY MOOD TODAY

6:00
7:00
8:00
9:00
10:00
11:00
12:00
1:00
2:00
3:00
4:00
5:00
6:00
7:00
8:00
8:00
9:00
10:00

○ BREAKFAST

○ _____

○ _____

VOTE ☆☆☆☆☆

○ LUNCH

○ _____

○ _____

VOTE ☆☆☆☆☆

○ DINNER

○ _____

○ _____

VOTE ☆☆☆☆☆

To Do list

Great things

NEVER came

from

Comfort zones ➤

WATER TRACKER
16 GLASSES OF WATER EACH DAY (1 GALLON)

COUNTDOWN

30 29
28 27 26 25 24 23 22
21 20 19 18 17 16 15
14 13 12 11 10 9 8
7 6 5 4 3 2 1

GOOD MORNING!

Shopping List:

MY MOOD TODAY

6:00 _____
7:00 _____
8:00 _____
9:00 _____
10:00 _____
11:00 _____
12:00 _____
1:00 _____
2:00 _____
3:00 _____
4:00 _____
5:00 _____
6:00 _____
7:00 _____
8:00 _____
8:00 _____
9:00 _____
10:00 _____

◯ BREAKFAST

◯ _____

◯ _____

VOTE ☆☆☆☆☆

◯ LUNCH

◯ _____

◯ _____

VOTE ☆☆☆☆☆

◯ DINNER

◯ _____

◯ _____

VOTE ☆☆☆☆☆

To Do list

WATER TRACKER
16 GLASSES OF WATER EACH DAY (1 GALLON)

I can
and
I will
WATCH ME

WEEKLY RESULTS

WEEK [1] [2] [3] [4]

WEIGHT _____

LOST WEIGHT _____

50%

WEEKLY GOALS

○ _____

○ _____

○ _____

CHECK YOUR GOALS FOR THE PAST WEEK. ARE YOU SATISFIED?
GIVE YOURSELF AN HONEST RATING ON A SCALE OF 1 TO 10.

_____
_____
_____

WHAT DID YOU DO AND WHAT COULD YOU BETTER?

_____
_____
_____

- FOR THE NEXT WEEK -

TO DO LIST

☐ _____
☐ _____
☐ _____
☐ _____
☐ _____
☐ _____
☐ _____
☐ _____
☐ _____

NOTES

_____
_____
_____
_____
_____
_____
_____

TOP 3 PRIORITIES

○ _____

○ _____

○ _____

Great things
NEVER came
from
Comfort zones

COUNTDOWN

(30) (29)
(28) (27) (26) (25) (24) (23) (22)
(21) (20) (19) (18) (17) (16) (15)
(14) (13) (12) (11) (10) (9) (8)
(7) (6) (5) (4) (3) (2) (1)

Good Morning!

MY MOOD TODAY

6:00 _____
7:00 _____
8:00 _____
9:00 _____
10:00 _____
11:00 _____
12:00 _____
1:00 _____
2:00 _____
3:00 _____
4:00 _____
5:00 _____
6:00 _____
7:00 _____
8:00 _____
8:00 _____
9:00 _____
10:00 _____

○ BREAKFAST

○ _____

○ _____

VOTE ☆☆☆☆☆

○ LUNCH

○ _____

○ _____

VOTE ☆☆☆☆☆

○ DINNER

○ _____

○ _____

VOTE ☆☆☆☆☆

Shopping List:

☐ _____
☐ _____
☐ _____
☐ _____
☐ _____
☐ _____
☐ _____
☐ _____
☐ _____
☐ _____

To Do List

☐ _____
☐ _____
☐ _____
☐ _____
☐ _____
☐ _____
☐ _____
☐ _____
☐ _____
☐ _____

IF YOU BELIEVE IN YOURSELF ANYTHING IS POSSIBLE.

WATER TRACKER

16 GLASSES OF WATER EACH DAY (1 GALLON)

COUNTDOWN

30 29
28 27 26 25 24 23 22
21 20 19 18 17 16 15
14 13 12 11 10 9 8
7 6 5 4 3 2 1

GOOD MORNING!

MY MOOD TODAY

6:00
7:00
8:00
9:00
10:00
11:00
12:00
1:00
2:00
3:00
4:00
5:00
6:00
7:00
8:00
8:00
9:00
10:00

◯ BREAKFAST
◯ _____
◯ _____
VOTE ☆☆☆☆☆

◯ LUNCH
◯ _____
◯ _____
VOTE ☆☆☆☆☆

◯ DINNER
◯ _____
◯ _____
VOTE ☆☆☆☆☆

Shopping List:

☐
☐
☐
☐
☐
☐
☐
☐
☐
☐

To Do list

☐
☐
☐
☐
☐
☐
☐
☐
☐
☐

WATER TRACKER
16 GLASSES OF WATER EACH DAY (1 GALLON)

Discipline is choosing between *what you want* NOW and *what you want* MOST
Abraham Lincoln

150

COUNTDOWN

30 29
28 27 26 25 24 23 22
21 20 19 18 17 16 15
14 13 12 11 10 9 8
7 6 5 4 3 2 1

GOOD MORNING!

MY MOOD TODAY

6:00
7:00
8:00
9:00
10:00
11:00
12:00
1:00
2:00
3:00
4:00
5:00
6:00
7:00
8:00
8:00
9:00
10:00

○ BREAKFAST
○
○
VOTE ☆☆☆☆☆

○ LUNCH
○
○
VOTE ☆☆☆☆☆

○ DINNER
○
○
VOTE ☆☆☆☆☆

Shopping List:

☐
☐
☐
☐
☐
☐
☐
☐
☐
☐
☐

To Do list

☐
☐
☐
☐
☐
☐
☐
☐
☐
☐
☐

IF IT IS IMPORTANT TO
YOU, YOU WILL FIND A
WAY. IF NOT, YOU WILL
FIND AN EXCUSE.

Ryan Blair

WATER TRACKER
16 GLASSES OF WATER EACH DAY (1 GALLON)

COUNTDOWN

30 29
28 27 26 25 24 23 22
21 20 19 18 17 16 15
14 13 12 11 10 9 8
7 6 5 4 3 2 1

GOOD MORNING!

MY MOOD TODAY

6:00 _____
7:00 _____
8:00 _____
9:00 _____
10:00 _____
11:00 _____
12:00 _____
1:00 _____
2:00 _____
3:00 _____
4:00 _____
5:00 _____
6:00 _____
7:00 _____
8:00 _____
8:00 _____
9:00 _____
10:00 _____

○ BREAKFAST _____
○ _____
○ _____
VOTE ☆☆☆☆☆

○ LUNCH _____
○ _____
○ _____
VOTE ☆☆☆☆☆

○ DINNER _____
○ _____
○ _____
VOTE ☆☆☆☆☆

Shopping List:
☐ _____
☐ _____
☐ _____
☐ _____
☐ _____
☐ _____
☐ _____
☐ _____
☐ _____
☐ _____

To Do list
☐ _____
☐ _____
☐ _____
☐ _____
☐ _____
☐ _____
☐ _____
☐ _____

Do something **today** that your **future** *self* will **thank** you for

WATER TRACKER

16 GLASSES OF WATER EACH DAY (1 GALLON)

COUNTDOWN

30 29
28 27 26 25 24 23 22
21 20 19 18 17 16 15
14 13 12 11 10 9 8
7 6 5 4 3 2 1

GOOD MORNING!

Shopping List:

☐
☐
☐
☐
☐
☐
☐
☐
☐
☐
☐

MY MOOD TODAY

6:00
7:00
8:00
9:00
10:00
11:00
12:00
1:00
2:00
3:00
4:00
5:00
6:00
7:00
8:00
8:00
9:00
10:00

○ BREAKFAST _____

○ _____

○ _____

VOTE ☆☆☆☆☆

○ LUNCH _____

○ _____

○ _____

VOTE ☆☆☆☆☆

○ DINNER _____

○ _____

○ _____

VOTE ☆☆☆☆☆

To Do List

☐
☐
☐
☐
☐
☐
☐
☐
☐
☐
☐
☐

I am not what happened to me, I am what I chose to become.

Carl Jung

WATER TRACKER

16 GLASSES OF WATER EACH DAY (1 GALLON)

COUNTDOWN

30 29
28 27 26 25 24 23 22
21 20 19 18 17 16 15
14 13 12 11 10 9 8
7 6 5 4 3 2 1

GOOD MORNING!

MY MOOD TODAY

6:00
7:00
8:00
9:00
10:00
11:00
12:00
1:00
2:00
3:00
4:00
5:00
6:00
7:00
8:00
8:00
9:00
10:00

○ BREAKFAST
○ _____
○ _____

VOTE ☆☆☆☆☆

○ LUNCH
○ _____
○ _____

VOTE ☆☆☆☆☆

○ DINNER
○ _____
○ _____

VOTE ☆☆☆☆☆

Shopping List:

To Do list

WATER TRACKER
16 GLASSES OF WATER EACH DAY (1 GALLON)

Your are
What you do
not
what you say
you will do

COUNTDOWN

30 29 28 27 26 25 24 23 22 21 20 19 18 17 16 15 14 13 12 11 10 9 8 7 6 5 4 3 2 1

GOOD MORNING!

MY MOOD TODAY

6:00 _____
7:00 _____
8:00 _____
9:00 _____
10:00 _____
11:00 _____
12:00 _____
1:00 _____
2:00 _____
3:00 _____
4:00 _____
5:00 _____
6:00 _____
7:00 _____
8:00 _____
8:00 _____
9:00 _____
10:00 _____

○ BREAKFAST _____
○ _____
○ _____
VOTE ☆☆☆☆☆

○ LUNCH _____
○ _____
○ _____
VOTE ☆☆☆☆☆

○ DINNER _____
○ _____
○ _____
VOTE ☆☆☆☆☆

Shopping List:
☐
☐
☐
☐
☐
☐
☐
☐
☐
☐

To Do list
☐
☐
☐
☐
☐
☐
☐
☐

Hard work beats talent when talent doesn't work hard.

Tim Notke

WATER TRACKER
16 GLASSES OF WATER EACH DAY (1 GALLON)

155

WEEKLY RESULTS

WEEK ① ② ③ ④

75%

WEIGHT _____

LOST WEIGHT _____

WEEKLY GOALS

○ _____

○ _____

○ _____

CHECK YOUR GOALS FOR THE PAST WEEK. ARE YOU SATISFIED?
GIVE YOURSELF AN HONEST RATING ON A SCALE OF 1 TO 10.

_____
_____
_____

WHAT DID YOU DO AND WHAT COULD YOU BETTER?

_____
_____
_____
_____

- FOR THE NEXT WEEK -

TO DO LIST

☐ _____
☐ _____
☐ _____
☐ _____
☐ _____
☐ _____
☐ _____
☐ _____
☐ _____

NOTES

_____
_____
_____
_____
_____
_____
_____
_____

TOP 3 PRIORITIES

○ _____
○ _____
○ _____

LOVE THE LIFE YOU LIVE.
LIVE THE LIFE YOU LOVE.

Bob Marley

COUNTDOWN

30 29
28 27 26 25 24 23 22
21 20 19 18 17 16 15
14 13 12 11 10 9 8
7 6 5 4 3 2 1

Good Morning!

MY MOOD TODAY

6:00
7:00
8:00
9:00
10:00
11:00
12:00
1:00
2:00
3:00
4:00
5:00
6:00
7:00
8:00
8:00
9:00
10:00

○ BREAKFAST

○
○
○

VOTE ☆☆☆☆☆

○ LUNCH

○
○

VOTE ☆☆☆☆☆

○ DINNER

○
○

VOTE ☆☆☆☆☆

Shopping List:

To Do List

DOUBT KILLS MORE DREAMS THAN FAILURE EVER WILL.

Suzy Kassem

WATER TRACKER

16 GLASSES OF WATER EACH DAY (1 GALLON)

157

COUNTDOWN

30 29
28 27 26 25 24 23 22
21 20 19 18 17 16 15
14 13 12 11 10 9 8
7 6 5 4 3 2 1

GOOD MORNING!

MY MOOD TODAY

6:00
7:00
8:00
9:00
10:00
11:00
12:00
1:00
2:00
3:00
4:00
5:00
6:00
7:00
8:00
8:00
9:00
10:00

○ BREAKFAST

○
○
VOTE ☆☆☆☆☆

○ LUNCH

○
○
VOTE ☆☆☆☆☆

○ DINNER

○
○
VOTE ☆☆☆☆☆

Shopping List:

☐
☐
☐
☐
☐
☐
☐
☐
☐

To Do List

☐
☐
☐
☐
☐
☐
☐
☐
☐
☐

WATER TRACKER

16 GLASSES OF WATER EACH DAY (1 GALLON)

DON'T STOP WHEN YOU ARE TIRED. STOP WHEN YOU ARE DONE.

COUNTDOWN

30 29 28 27 26 25 24 23 22 21 20 19 18 17 16 15 14 13 12 11 10 9 8 7 6 5 4 3 2 1

GOOD MORNING!

MY MOOD TODAY

6:00 _____
7:00 _____
8:00 _____
9:00 _____
10:00 _____
11:00 _____
12:00 _____
1:00 _____
2:00 _____
3:00 _____
4:00 _____
5:00 _____
6:00 _____
7:00 _____
8:00 _____
8:00 _____
9:00 _____
10:00 _____

◯ BREAKFAST _____

◯ _____

◯ _____

VOTE ☆☆☆☆☆

◯ LUNCH _____

◯ _____

◯ _____

VOTE ☆☆☆☆☆

◯ DINNER _____

◯ _____

◯ _____

VOTE ☆☆☆☆☆

Shopping List:

☐
☐
☐
☐
☐
☐
☐
☐
☐
☐
☐

To Do list

☐
☐
☐
☐
☐
☐
☐
☐
☐
☐

WATER TRACKER

16 GLASSES OF WATER EACH DAY (1 GALLON)

A **Negative mind** will **NEVER** **GIVE YOU** a **Positive life**

COUNTDOWN

(30) (29)
(28) (27) (26) (25) (24) (23) (22)
(21) (20) (19) (18) (17) (16) (15)
(14) (13) (12) (11) (10) (9) (8)
(7) (6) (5) (4) (3) (2) (1)

GOOD MORNING!

MY MOOD TODAY

6:00 _____
7:00 _____
8:00 _____
9:00 _____
10:00 _____
11:00 _____
12:00 _____
1:00 _____
2:00 _____
3:00 _____
4:00 _____
5:00 _____
6:00 _____
7:00 _____
8:00 _____
8:00 _____
9:00 _____
10:00 _____

○ BREAKFAST
○ _____
○ _____
VOTE ☆☆☆☆☆

○ LUNCH
○ _____
○ _____
VOTE ☆☆☆☆☆

○ DINNER
○ _____
○ _____
VOTE ☆☆☆☆☆

Shopping List:

☐ _____
☐ _____
☐ _____
☐ _____
☐ _____
☐ _____
☐ _____
☐ _____
☐ _____
☐ _____

To Do List

☐ _____
☐ _____
☐ _____
☐ _____
☐ _____
☐ _____
☐ _____
☐ _____
☐ _____
☐ _____

WATER TRACKER

16 GLASSES OF WATER EACH DAY (1 GALLON)

DIFFICULT ROADS OFTEN LEAD TO BEAUTIFUL DESTINATIONS.

COUNTDOWN

30 29
28 27 26 25 24 23 22
21 20 19 18 17 16 15
14 13 12 11 10 9 8
7 6 5 4 3 2 1

GOOD MORNING!

Shopping List:

☐
☐
☐
☐
☐
☐
☐
☐
☐
☐

MY MOOD TODAY

6:00 _____
7:00 _____
8:00 _____
9:00 _____
10:00 _____
11:00 _____
12:00 _____
1:00 _____
2:00 _____
3:00 _____
4:00 _____
5:00 _____
6:00 _____
7:00 _____
8:00 _____
8:00 _____
9:00 _____
10:00 _____

○ BREAKFAST
○ _____
○ _____
VOTE ☆☆☆☆☆

○ LUNCH
○ _____
○ _____
VOTE ☆☆☆☆☆

○ DINNER
○ _____
○ _____
VOTE ☆☆☆☆☆

To Do list

☐
☐
☐
☐
☐
☐
☐
☐
☐

A RIVER CUTS THROUGH
ROCK, NOT BECAUSE
OF ITS POWER, BUT
BECAUSE OF ITS
PERSISTENCE.

Jim Watkins

WATER TRACKER
16 GLASSES OF WATER EACH DAY (1 GALLON)

COUNTDOWN

30 29
28 27 26 25 24 23 22
21 20 19 18 17 16 15
14 13 12 11 10 9 8
7 6 5 4 3 2 1

GOOD MORNING!

MY MOOD TODAY

6:00 _____
7:00 _____
8:00 _____
9:00 _____
10:00 _____
11:00 _____
12:00 _____
1:00 _____
2:00 _____
3:00 _____
4:00 _____
5:00 _____
6:00 _____
7:00 _____
8:00 _____
8:00 _____
9:00 _____
10:00 _____

○ BREAKFAST _____
○ _____
○ _____
VOTE ☆☆☆☆☆

○ LUNCH _____
○ _____
○ _____
VOTE ☆☆☆☆☆

○ DINNER _____
○ _____
○ _____
VOTE ☆☆☆☆☆

Shopping List:

☐ _____
☐ _____
☐ _____
☐ _____
☐ _____
☐ _____
☐ _____
☐ _____
☐ _____
☐ _____

To Do list

☐ _____
☐ _____
☐ _____
☐ _____
☐ _____
☐ _____
☐ _____
☐ _____
☐ _____
☐ _____
☐ _____

WATER TRACKER
16 GLASSES OF WATER EACH DAY (1 GALLON)

Motivation is what gets you started.
Habit is what keeps you going.
Jim Rohn

162

COUNTDOWN

30 29
28 27 26 25 24 23 22
21 20 19 18 17 16 15
14 13 12 11 10 9 8
7 6 5 4 3 2 1

GOOD MORNING!

Shopping List:

MY MOOD TODAY

6:00 _____
7:00 _____
8:00 _____
9:00 _____
10:00 _____
11:00 _____
12:00 _____
1:00 _____
2:00 _____
3:00 _____
4:00 _____
5:00 _____
6:00 _____
7:00 _____
8:00 _____
8:00 _____
9:00 _____
10:00 _____

◯ BREAKFAST _____
◯ _____
◯ _____
VOTE ☆☆☆☆☆

◯ LUNCH _____
◯ _____
◯ _____
VOTE ☆☆☆☆☆

◯ DINNER _____
◯ _____
◯ _____
VOTE ☆☆☆☆☆

To Do List

WATER TRACKER
16 GLASSES OF WATER EACH DAY (1 GALLON)

INHALE
love
EXHALE
gratitude

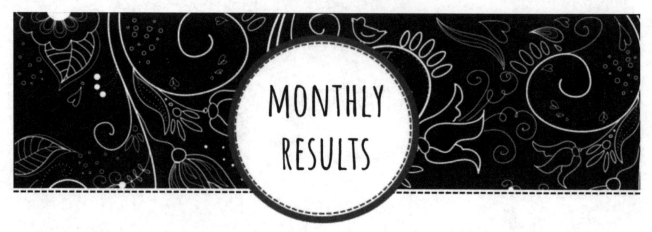

MONTHLY RESULTS

CONGRATULATIONS, YOU HAVE COMPLETED YOUR DEXOTIFICATION JOURNEY!

WEIGHT _____

LOST WEIGHT _____

100%

MONTHLY GOALS

○ _____

○ _____

○ _____

HOW DO YOU FEEL ABOUT YOUR PHYSICAL AND MENTAL STATE NOW?.

_____

_____

_____

_____

COMPARE YOUR ANSWER TO THE GOALS YOU WROTE A MONTH AGO.
ARE YOU SATISFIED WITH YOUR RESULTS?

_____

_____

_____

_____

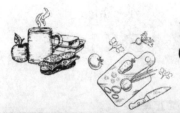

Results can only change when we change our consistent actions and make them habits.
Billy Cox

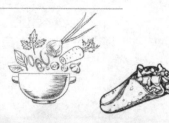

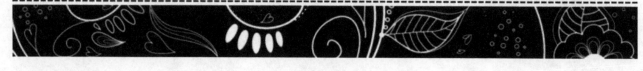

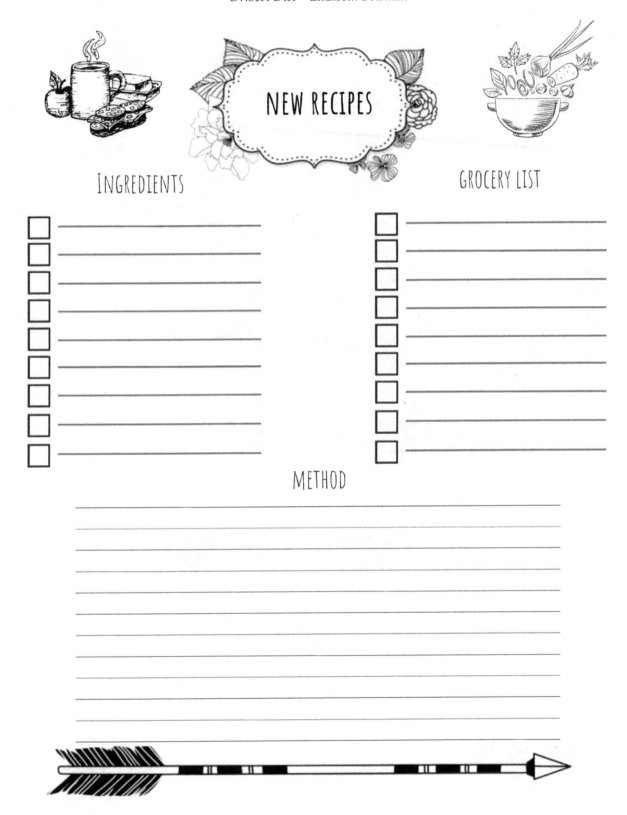

NEW RECIPES

INGREDIENTS

- [ ] _____
- [ ] _____
- [ ] _____
- [ ] _____
- [ ] _____
- [ ] _____
- [ ] _____
- [ ] _____
- [ ] _____

GROCERY LIST

- [ ] _____
- [ ] _____
- [ ] _____
- [ ] _____
- [ ] _____
- [ ] _____
- [ ] _____
- [ ] _____
- [ ] _____

METHOD

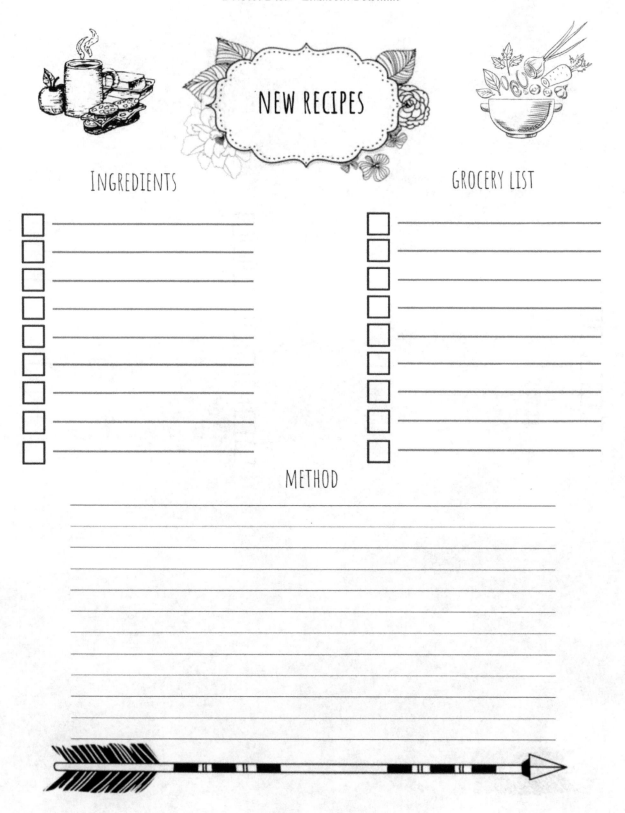

NEW RECIPES

INGREDIENTS

- ☐ _____
- ☐ _____
- ☐ _____
- ☐ _____
- ☐ _____
- ☐ _____
- ☐ _____
- ☐ _____
- ☐ _____

GROCERY LIST

- ☐ _____
- ☐ _____
- ☐ _____
- ☐ _____
- ☐ _____
- ☐ _____
- ☐ _____
- ☐ _____
- ☐ _____

METHOD

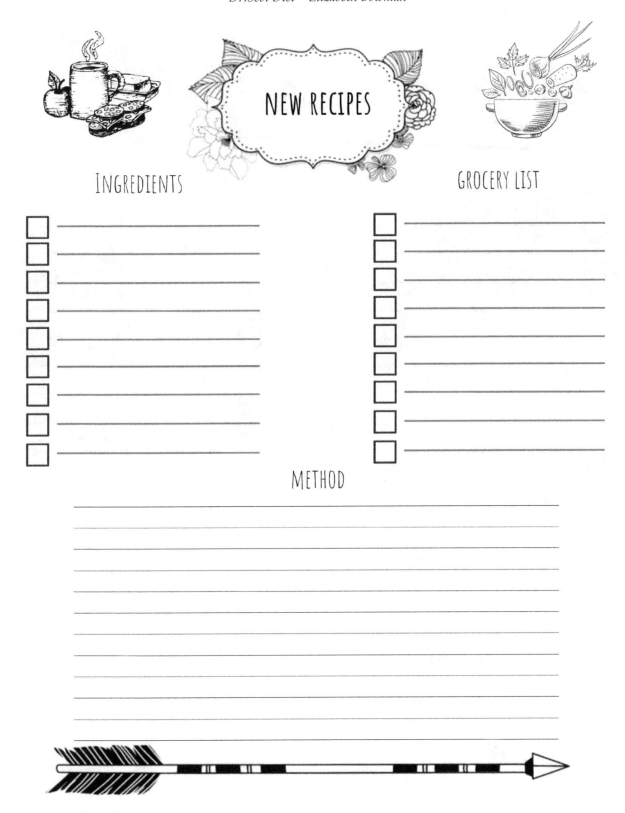

NEW RECIPES

INGREDIENTS

- [ ] _____
- [ ] _____
- [ ] _____
- [ ] _____
- [ ] _____
- [ ] _____
- [ ] _____
- [ ] _____
- [ ] _____

GROCERY LIST

- [ ] _____
- [ ] _____
- [ ] _____
- [ ] _____
- [ ] _____
- [ ] _____
- [ ] _____
- [ ] _____

METHOD

_____
_____
_____
_____
_____
_____
_____
_____
_____
_____
_____

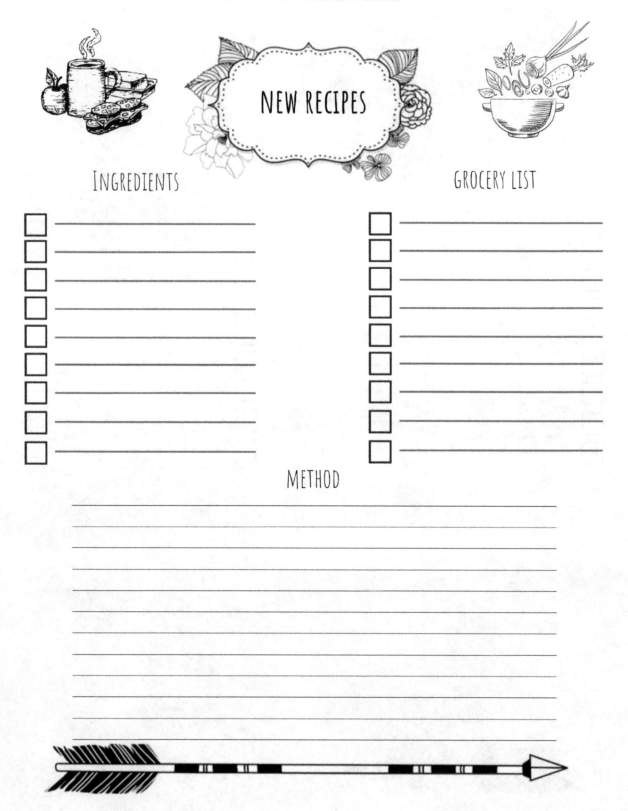

NEW RECIPES

INGREDIENTS

- ☐ _____
- ☐ _____
- ☐ _____
- ☐ _____
- ☐ _____
- ☐ _____
- ☐ _____
- ☐ _____
- ☐ _____

GROCERY LIST

- ☐ _____
- ☐ _____
- ☐ _____
- ☐ _____
- ☐ _____
- ☐ _____
- ☐ _____
- ☐ _____

METHOD

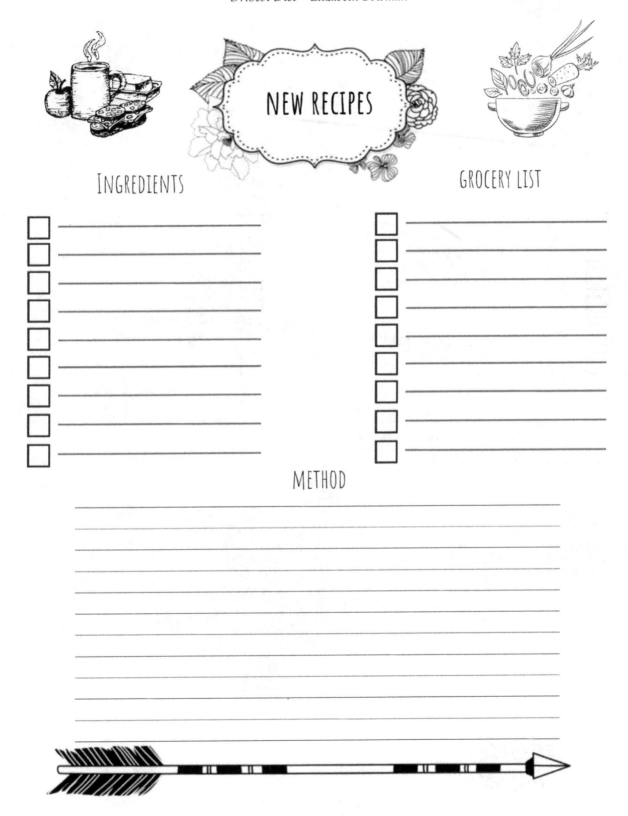

NEW RECIPES

INGREDIENTS

- [ ]
- [ ]
- [ ]
- [ ]
- [ ]
- [ ]
- [ ]
- [ ]
- [ ]

GROCERY LIST

- [ ]
- [ ]
- [ ]
- [ ]
- [ ]
- [ ]
- [ ]
- [ ]
- [ ]

METHOD

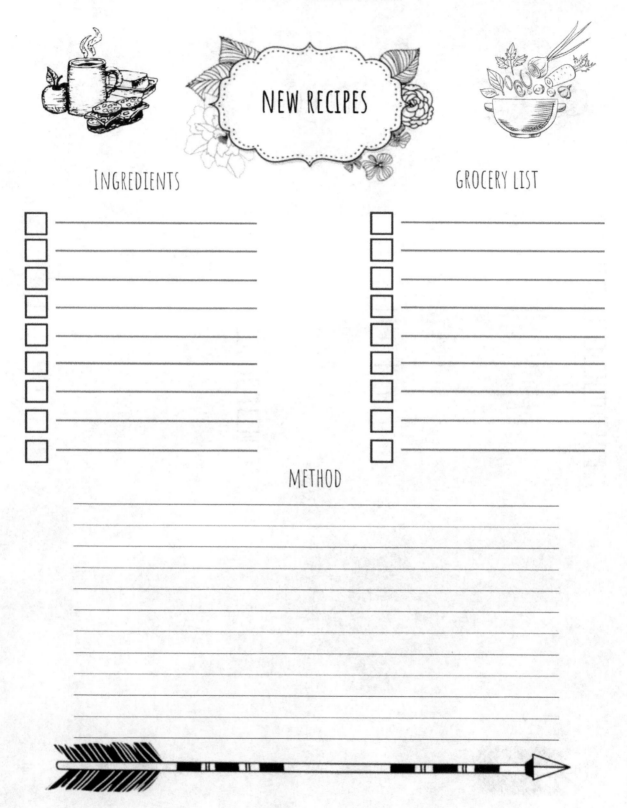

NEW RECIPES

INGREDIENTS

- [ ] _____
- [ ] _____
- [ ] _____
- [ ] _____
- [ ] _____
- [ ] _____
- [ ] _____
- [ ] _____
- [ ] _____

GROCERY LIST

- [ ] _____
- [ ] _____
- [ ] _____
- [ ] _____
- [ ] _____
- [ ] _____
- [ ] _____
- [ ] _____
- [ ] _____

METHOD

_____
_____
_____
_____
_____
_____
_____
_____
_____
_____
_____

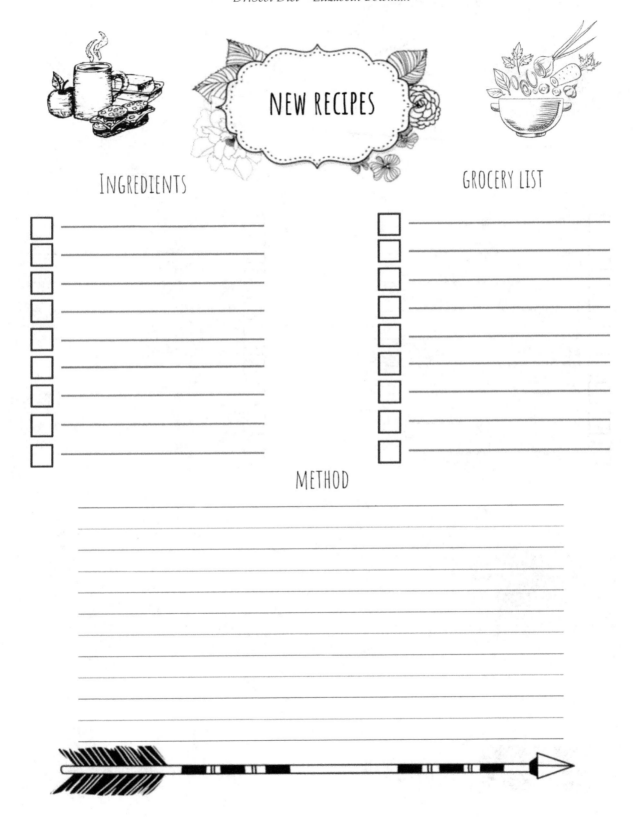

NEW RECIPES

INGREDIENTS

- ☐ _____
- ☐ _____
- ☐ _____
- ☐ _____
- ☐ _____
- ☐ _____
- ☐ _____
- ☐ _____
- ☐ _____

GROCERY LIST

- ☐ _____
- ☐ _____
- ☐ _____
- ☐ _____
- ☐ _____
- ☐ _____
- ☐ _____
- ☐ _____
- ☐ _____

METHOD

_____
_____
_____
_____
_____
_____
_____
_____
_____
_____
_____
_____

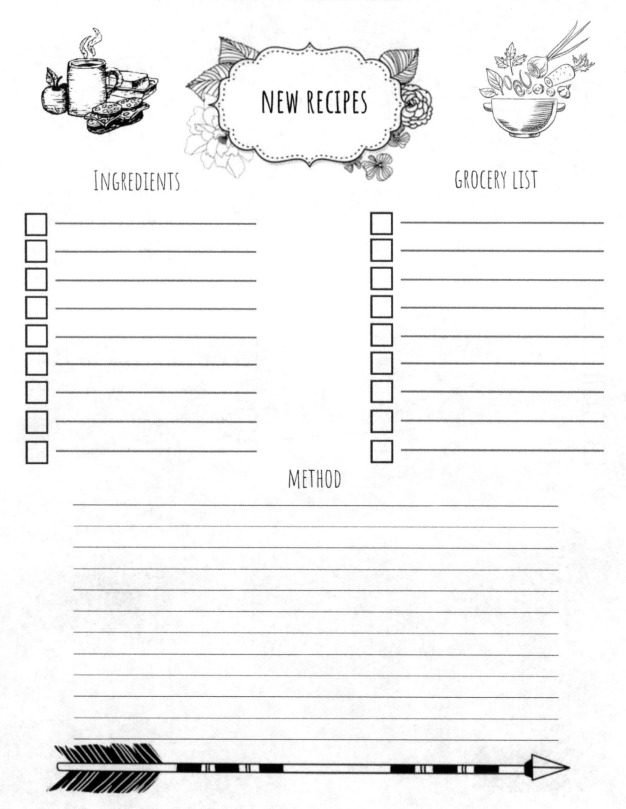

NEW RECIPES

INGREDIENTS

- [ ] _____
- [ ] _____
- [ ] _____
- [ ] _____
- [ ] _____
- [ ] _____
- [ ] _____
- [ ] _____
- [ ] _____

GROCERY LIST

- [ ] _____
- [ ] _____
- [ ] _____
- [ ] _____
- [ ] _____
- [ ] _____
- [ ] _____
- [ ] _____
- [ ] _____

METHOD

_____
_____
_____
_____
_____
_____
_____
_____
_____
_____
_____

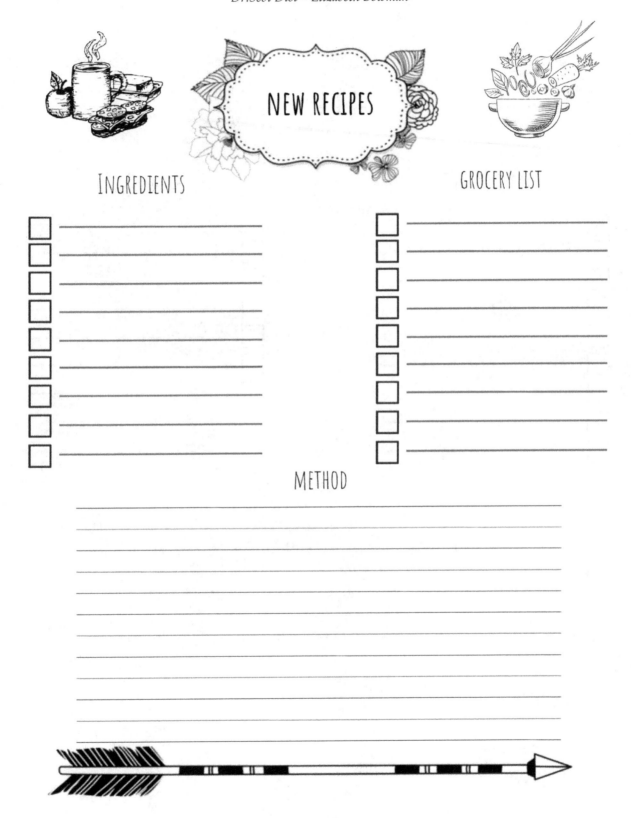

NEW RECIPES

INGREDIENTS

- [ ] _____
- [ ] _____
- [ ] _____
- [ ] _____
- [ ] _____
- [ ] _____
- [ ] _____
- [ ] _____
- [ ] _____

GROCERY LIST

- [ ] _____
- [ ] _____
- [ ] _____
- [ ] _____
- [ ] _____
- [ ] _____
- [ ] _____
- [ ] _____
- [ ] _____

METHOD

_____
_____
_____
_____
_____
_____
_____
_____
_____
_____
_____
_____
_____
_____

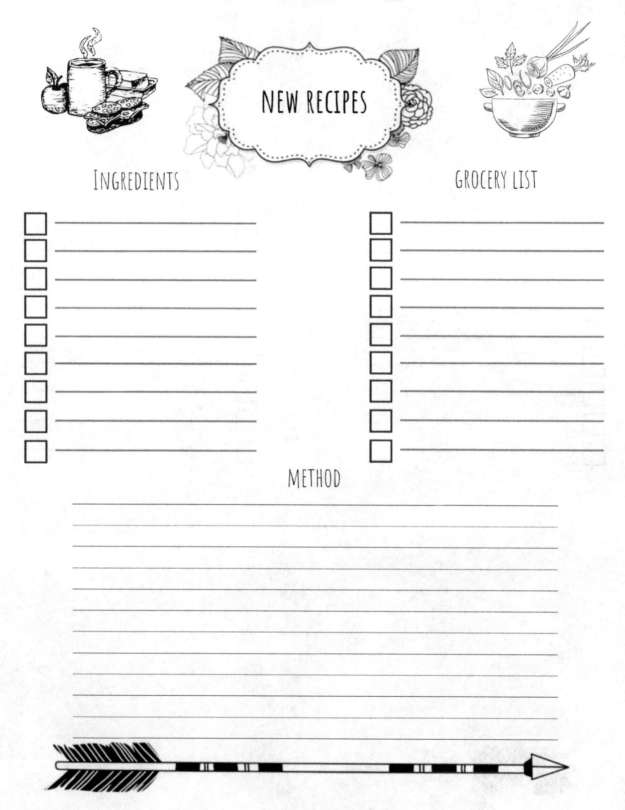

NEW RECIPES

INGREDIENTS

- ☐ _____
- ☐ _____
- ☐ _____
- ☐ _____
- ☐ _____
- ☐ _____
- ☐ _____
- ☐ _____
- ☐ _____

GROCERY LIST

- ☐ _____
- ☐ _____
- ☐ _____
- ☐ _____
- ☐ _____
- ☐ _____
- ☐ _____
- ☐ _____

METHOD

_____
_____
_____
_____
_____
_____
_____
_____
_____
_____
_____

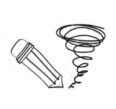
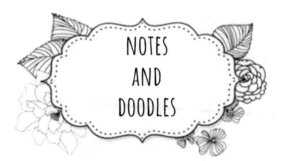

NOTES
AND
DOODLES

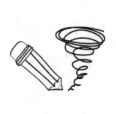
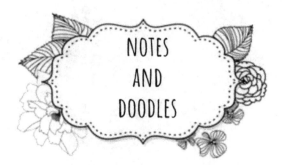

NOTES AND DOODLES

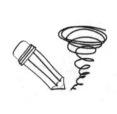
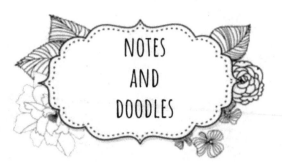

NOTES
AND
DOODLES

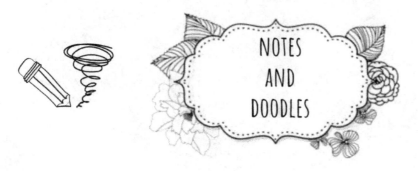

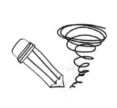
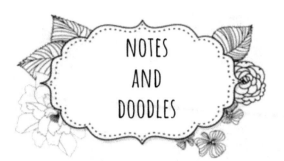

NOTES
AND
DOODLES

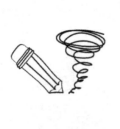
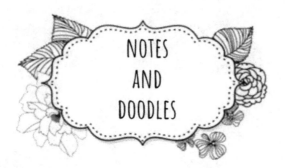

NOTES
AND
DOODLES

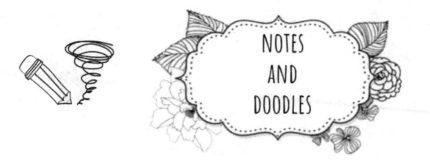

NOTES AND DOODLES

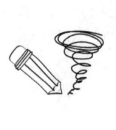 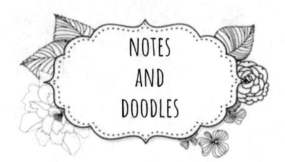 

NOTES
AND
DOODLES

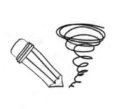

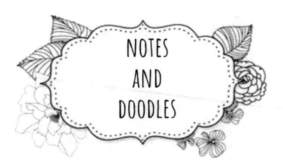

NOTES
AND
DOODLES

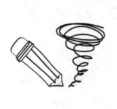
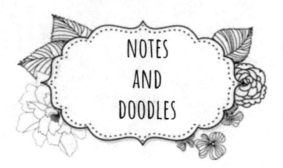

NOTES AND DOODLES

REMEMBER!

You'll be able to fill out your daily plan directly in the book or download a printable version at the link you see below to use the planner all year round as well.

https://ebowmanwriter.wixsite.com/doctorsebi

Journal created with the collaboration of **www.101planners.com**